Quiet Mind
Warrior Spirit

Conscious self-defense for everyday life

Quiet Mind Warrior Spirit

Conscious self-defense for everyday life

Lila Reyna

Bascom Hill Publishing Group

Bascom Hill Publishing Group
212 3rd Avenue North, Suite 570
Minneapolis, MN 55401
612.455.2293
www.bascomhillpublishing.com

ISBN - 978-1-935098-08-9
ISBN - 1-935098-08-x
LCCN - 2008938821

Book sales for North America and international:
Itasca Books, 3501 Highway 100 South, Suite 220
Minneapolis, MN 55416
Phone: 952.345.4488 (toll free 1.800.901.3480)
Fax: 952.920.0541; email to orders@itascabooks.com

Cover Design by Wes Moore
Typeset by Peggy LeTrent
Photography by Mike Bringolf

Printed in the United States of America

BASCOM HILL
PUBLISHING GROUP

Disclaimer

The physical self-defense techniques, applications of Psychosymmetrolysis, personal experiences of the author, and the stories of other individuals included in this book are for interest purposes only.

The martial art techniques presented have been used and monitored in many workshops and real-life applications. No harm has come to any participant as a result. However, implementing the personal guidelines listed in this book is potentially dangerous and could cause serious injury or death without the proper instruction and supervision from a trained professional. It is important to act sensibly and responsibly when undertaking any physical or introspectively challenging work.

Any application of the techniques and approaches in this book remains at the reader's own risk, and the authors and publishers disclaim any liability arising directly or indirectly from their use.

Know yourself and you will win all battles.
—Sun Tzo

Contents

Acknowledgements   xiii

Introduction   1

CHAPTER ONE   3
Between a Mess and a Miracle
    Beginning the journey of self-appreciation

CHAPTER TWO   13
Survival: Learning to Live
    Psychosymmetrolysis in our daily life

CHAPTER THREE   23
Knowledge is Prevention: Awareness of the Assailant
    Understanding crime assailants

CHAPTER FOUR   33
Spiritual Pretension
    Facing our "truths" and finding purpose

CHAPTER FIVE   45
The Enemy Within: Domestic Violence
    Restoring self and knowing you are not alone

CHAPTER SIX   57
Understanding the Cycle of Abuse
    Ways in which we harm ourselves

CHAPTER SEVEN   65
How Far Do We Go?
    Healing from the inside out

CHAPTER EIGHT   73
The Mind: Credible or Crazy?
    The mind and our emotions

CHAPTER NINE   93
The Body as a Weapon
    Effective techniques for physical self-defense

CHAPTER TEN   109
The Main Target Areas
    Utilizing the vulnerable points of the body

CHAPTER ELEVEN   121
Safety and Sanity
    Balancing the mind, body, and spirit

CHAPTER TWELVE   133
Take Charge of Your Life
    Empower yourself today

CHAPTER THIRTEEN   147
The Key to Awareness: Balancing Intuition and Logic
    The essence of self-protection

References   161

Resources   163

Personal Notes   171

About the Author   173

Acknowledgements and Thanks

Many inspiring people were instrumental in the creation of this book, either directly or indirectly. My thanks to the individuals who shared their personal stories, the incredible Circle of Friends who provide everlasting laughter, support and friendship, my editor Adryan Russ, and the dedicated ladies at the Domestic Violence and Sexual Assault Coalition.

A special thank you to...
My husband, Kwan Jahng Nym Tony, for his support and training;

My children, Ishaan and Chela, for their understanding and patience;

My oldest, Jim, for constantly "pushing my buttons" and challenging me to see beyond my "truths;"

Jill, for answering my endless stream of computer questions;

Dad and Mom (the most loving and dedicated grandparents) for helping make quiet writing time possible; and, of course,
Ondre, for believing in me and passing on the greatest gift: passion for life.

Do you take life too seriously?

Maybe it's time to lighten up and have some fun! Today is the only day we have. We can't do anything about the past and we don't know exactly what the future holds. Many people go through life with low self-esteem, feelings of inadequacies, or a focus on the negative. We search for happiness everywhere and, over the centuries, people have tried to hold on to the state of blissful perfection through all sorts of external means—through power, sex, drugs, crime, and the accumulation of petty things, but it doesn't keep.

Complete self-defense is a synthesis of the mind, body, and heart, which together create the synergy of empowerment. People who do well in life are often ordinary people who have developed skills that enable them to survive difficult times. Even if we have had a challenging childhood, adolescence, and/or adult life, every one of us has the ability to step out of the self-images and beliefs that have darkened our life. You have the ability to let go of the past and start—right here, right now—and enlarge your vision.

Training the physical body for self-defense is beneficial, but it is essential to exercise the mind—to keep it free and flowing in order to act quickly and instinctively in any situation. Many times the best self-protection can be laughter, or simply slowing down to appreciate what is around you and within you. For those suffering from illness, abuse, or loss, naturally there is a time for grievance; yet if we take anything too seriously we end up limiting ourselves with fears and other unforgiving self-created blocks, while allowing bountiful opportunities to pass by untouched.

Through martial arts and the natural healing art of Psychosymmetrolysis, my goal is to provide self-defense approaches that can be helpful in our ever-changing world. Although I have trained in martial arts since 1993, I do not define victorious self-defense by the possession or degree of a black belt. However, as a means of integrative prevention, it is important to have some understanding and knowledge of the physical realms of self-defense. We may not need to apply the physical aspect of defense daily, but our awareness is challenged each day while driving a car, during a conversation or confrontation with another, traveling in foreign countries or simply engaging in a child's infinite stream of unanswerable questions.

Whether you intend to use this book as a simple manual or read it cover to cover, what matters most is how you choose to apply and put into action the information that is most helpful to you. Whatever you are searching or not searching for, whatever your religion or belief, I have great respect for each individual's path. To have knowledge of the potential dangers we face daily, both external and internal, is the foundation of conscious self-defense. This heightened sense of awareness relieves the busy commotion of the mind and abandons the desire of ego, which, in turn, supports the awakening of mental, physical, and spiritual safety, success, and happiness.

Chapter 1

Between a Mess and a Miracle

A complex situation often develops from un-complex means not being understood.
—Ondre

By age twenty-six I was a well-seasoned veteran when it came to the experience of new age, holistic, and sometimes bizarre alternative methods of "living spiritually." I endured needle punctures, taps on the brain, abnormal body stretches, and leftover bruises from unruly past lives. Then there was the occasional touch so gentle that I opened my eyes in fear that the practitioner went to lunch, leaving me vulnerable and butt-naked on the table.

There were some exceptional practitioners who paid heed to the smallest details with genuine care, and I was open to any prospect that might resemble this method of healing. Practitioners came in all sizes and shapes and embraced a diversity of clothing trends. Some practitioners wore professional business suits with matching ties. They spoke with a self-confidence that sometimes threatened to alter my meticulously established views. The more natural-type practitioners were wrapped in loose-fitting, free-flowing, rayon fabrics with rainbow colors. In time I adjusted to the heavily twisted and cured dreadlocks that rested upon the heads of many of these innate healers. Another practitioner smiled continuously and tried her best to tell me what she thought I wanted to hear. This was confusing because, like anyone, I found it wonderful to affirm my successes, but little actual momentum transpired, except for the continual rescheduling of appointments. And, of course, there were those who found clothing optional and basically useless, but I had little contact with these excessively liberated, freewheeling types.

The reading of star alignments and psychic visits was a common occurrence during my deranged search for something—the something that, at that point, had no physical shape, no cerebral comprehension, or spiritual reception. There was no word to describe what I searched for, because I was not even sure of what it was I longed for. How is it that you know when something is missing, yet the something in the equation does not present itself? I'm not exceptionally skilled at math, but it doesn't take many smarts to realize when part of the equation is missing. I instinctively felt a gaping hole, as if there were a missing piece to this puzzle of life. I was led only by an inward, nagging feeling that was far from gentle. The missing variable had the power to turn me into a bottomless pit of streaming tears. Subtract a lack of self-love and faith, add a deep sense of guilt, and it equals the broken equation I had become. At its worst, my situation emulated a brightly lit candle whose flame expired, leaving only the ash-gray smoke evaporating into nothingness.

This feeling of nothingness or emptiness drove me to search with uncertain certainty for something out there; I was determined to find it. The result of my search would, I hoped, restore the missing variables. It sounds a simple solution to a complex equation, and I felt the something was close to me. I could feel it practically exhaling warm puffs of breath down my neck; it was right around the corner—I just knew it. The only problem was the numerous unpredictable corners, twists, and turns that presented themselves internally and externally. But I am happy to say that even in my most crazed and afflicted moments, while searching for this somethingness, I did refrain from accepting one practitioner's enthusiastic offer for a fecal reading.

In October 2000, I sat on a weather-beaten gray bench outside a small cottage in the serene Sierra Nevada Foothills. By now, familiarity had bred boredom and I sat shivering in the brisk autumn breeze contemplating how many coins I had wasted on previous psychic appointments.

Before I calculated the rising figure, the door swung open to reveal a man with black, stylishly slicked-back hair. He was neither fat nor slim, no dreadlocks, no fancy tie, and no shining mythical deity aura. He carried professionalism about him, and he had a kind smile. His intense liquid-brown eyes instantly and quite unexpectedly relaxed me into a sensation of spreading warmth like the springtime sun after a winter downpour. Just as this curious warmth flushed through my system, the man's presence seemed to prompt a sudden and sharp inhalation of cool evening air. The cold air passed through my nostrils and filled my chest. The most peculiar feeling overcame me. Could it be possible? Do I already know this man? I quickly rummaged through my jumbled memory of previous practitioners, therapists, hairstylists, doctors, dentists, garbage men, boyfriends, and a variety of sport coaches. I was confident that I never had an appointment with this natural healer and respected medium. Why did it feel that I knew him with the familiarity of a next-door neighbor or even my brother? I sat speechless.

On that day, it was not the wind that left me shivering, but a mass of untamed nerves shuddered with anticipation of a major life change. No, it wasn't as if I was going to get married. I am married. I wasn't getting divorced. I had already jumped from that sizzling frying pan once.

This was a life change more frightening and foreign to my consciousness. It was a combination of divorcing myself from fabricated truths that I had created and remarrying my self—with the developed commitment to appreciate and love myself. It may not sound that bad but, the process of seeking self-appreciation and self-protection can also feel like—forgive the image—a bloody can of gutted worms.

With a steaming hot mug cupped between my hands, I stared at Ondre. I was told that this man was a uniquely gifted natural healer who is recognized worldwide for being in the forefront of healing with energy, but he was far from my illusionary mind's eye of the older, mystical wizard. There was no majestic white beard resting upon his chest. There was no beard at all, no flowing golden velvet robe. Instead of holding the Harry Potter-like magic wand that I had envisioned and desperately needed, his hands held only a cup of Earl Gray tea.

I sipped my mint tea, swishing the herbal sweetness in my mouth. While contemplating what this middle-aged man, dressed casually in dark blue jeans and a crisp black collared shirt, could possibly do for me, I considered what imperative question I should ask first. Much to my astonishment, he began questioning me.

Ondre spoke with a hearty British accent. "What did you do this morning?"

I swallowed, feeling the hot tea slide down my throat, warming my insides and creating an embarrassing gurgle that echoed across my cramping intestines. I dearly hoped I wouldn't pass gas. "I took the kids to school," I replied, flicking the long strands of hair out of my eyes with a quick sweep of the hand, feeling agitated by this exceptionally plain question.

"No, before that," Ondre bluntly stated, but in a kind tone.

He sat patiently waiting for my memory to ignite. I stared at his polished black shoes while searching my suddenly empty and oblivious brain for any recollection of the morning.

He spoke quietly. "It was in the morning, right after you went to the bathroom."

No sooner did he speak these words then the mental picture burst through my mind. I saw myself board the bathroom scale, take note of my inflated weight and sink further into the painful realms of sadness. I sat up quickly and then drank another long sip of tea, hoping to drown out the vivid image. As I peered over the rim of the mug, I saw Ondre nod his head up and down slowly, which I later learned is a sure indicator of further discussions to come. *No way, I do not consider myself depressed. Even with the daily drama I am living, I am far too optimistic. Don't forget, I said to myself, disregarding any humble qualities, I am a martial artist. I not only practice external disabling techniques, I am constantly building internal strength and power—Ki energy…no, I definitely could not be someone to fall into any level of depression.* In that overly prideful and arrogant moment (I had many more to come), I convinced myself that I could rest assured, for I certainly was not a victim of any silly internal weakness or illness. No way, I thought to myself again, depression could not possibly be part of my path…or could it?

A curious feature of depression is that it is possible to be depressed and not even know it. I think, perhaps, I was living proof of this sad fact. People often know how to mask their feelings and hide them, not only from others but, from themselves as well. If you can smile when feeling down, then others may think you are doing fine, but depression can't stay hidden within you without eventually showing through as a physical condition, mental illness, or spiritual constipation. I will spare you unnecessary visuals, but I must say that my *stuff* was stuck, condensed, and compacted. My collection of internal anger and frustrations caused massive self-induced hemorrhoids. I itched for relief from the throbbing pain of self-hatred and perfectionism from which molded the destructive bulge of depression.

> **Emptiness, anger and depression can find anyone, anywhere...if we let it. Depression is a state of mind and, for many, an excuse. It can be a selfish act, focused on the person and what he or she wants and needs.**

Although depression often goes undetected and untreated, it is estimated that between two and four percent of the general population suffers from clinical depression. In hard figures this means that during the course of a year, 17.5 million Americans suffer from depression. (BJS, 2007)

Many different symptoms make up the condition we label as depression; sadness is only one of them. Everyone feels sad now and then, such as when the family pet dies or a romantic partnership breaks apart, but some people are unaware of the sadness that lingers inside. If allowed to become "familiar," it then becomes accepted, in a way, as part of who we are. This can make it easy to disregard depression, overlook it or just plain deny it. There are many different symptoms; the degree of these symptoms in your life determines whether or not you are suffering from depression.

Some symptoms of depression are: feeling punished; a sense of failure, guilt, lack of energy, crying, poor appetite, weight loss, lack of libido, difficulty in making decisions, and self-criticism. Depression has been called "the common cold of mental health." Symptoms can be physical, behavioral, and emotional, with contributing factors stemming from environmental, interpersonal, biological, diet/exercise, and spiritual features. If you know how to "put on a happy face" when you're feeling down, then you are good at hiding emotion. Be careful not to fool yourself.

After the appointment with Ondre, I felt like a huge weight had lifted. A veil still covered my face, but I felt I could see through it, at least partially, as he proceeded to amaze me and awaken my mind. At one point, he slowly placed his left hand four inches above my right shoulder and, with caring concern, asked if I had been in a skiing accident about twelve years earlier. The dull ache and partially limited use of my shoulder was indeed a daily reminder of my horrific ski crash and, yes, I confirmed it was exactly twelve years ago. Ondre continued to hold his hand four inches above my shoulder for the next three minutes. As he did, I felt a rush of warmth and a slight prickly feeling spread, first down my arm and then throughout my body. I became relaxed and comfortable to a point that I didn't notice Ondre remove his hand until he resumed his sitting position.

Many uncertainties and questions shot through my head as if firing an automatic pistol at a fast moving target. *Is this possible? Are there really such things as miracles? What is healing energy? Where does it come from? Is there really something out there beyond us?* In response to my logical mind, I tried my best to feel any reminiscence of pain remaining in my shoulder, but to no avail. Incredibly, my shoulder was and is, to this day, free from pain and injury. But the mind, well, let me just say that it takes a bit longer to undo, redirect and heal that fist-size hunk of gray matter!

The session covered far more than I fathomed possible, taking some twists and turns that continued to challenge my wits long after I left.

As I walked to the door Ondre quietly said, "You have one more question...what is it?" He smiled compassionately, not so much with his lips, but when I looked into the depth of his eyes it was as if, for just a moment, I saw the beauty of myself mirrored back at me. It was a surprising but welcome reflection. The reflection I most frequently saw in a mirror was the contorted and twisted self-image, much like those "fun houses" at the county fair that deform you beyond recognition.

My mind raced with personal questions and about his whereabouts, wealth of information, and exceptional accuracy. One question burned in my heart with an undeniable passion and, after years of searching, finally, I knew he was the right one to ask. In my meek attempt to inquire if he would be my teacher, only a shy thank you squeaked out, flushing my pink cheeks a shade darker. Quickly I lowered my eyes and shuffled through the cottage door to meet the cool evening air with the awful and familiar feeling of anger. Again, I had not been brave enough to ask for what I wanted.

"Just remember," he said in a compassionate, matter-of-fact tone before I was out of hearing distance, "the answer is yes."

I left the cottage visibly shaking and barely able to grasp the steering wheel of the car. Shocked that he had answered my unspoken question and from the mind-boggling session, the sudden screech of tires from the vehicle ahead of me jolted my consciousness into the present with a frightening clarity. I gripped the steering wheel, giving it a sharp jerk in the hope of avoiding a collision with a shaggy black and white dog that seemed to appear out of nowhere. He hobbled across the road on three legs with great difficulty. I slowed down and came to a complete stop. Looking at the dog made me thankful for my own two intact legs. With a heavy head and large drooping eyes, he struggled to look up at me through the blinding headlights. I spoke out loud as if he might hear me. "I'm sorry, dog, go on now and safely get across the road. Thank you for reminding me that whatever kind of mess I am in, there is always someone worse off. You are quite beautiful despite your misery."

Even though I felt confused, mentally rattled, and emotionally hung, that evening helped me make some life-changing choices. On that day, I was offered a gift. I was presented with an opportunity to once again believe in myself; it was the gift of hope. This was an end to many self-made fantasies as well as a fresh beginning in the light of truth, self-protection, and survival.

Chapter 2

Survival: Learning to Live

The human being is part of the whole, called by us the universe, a part limited in time and space. We experience ourselves, our thoughts, and feelings as something separate from the rest, a kind of optical delusion of consciousness. This delusion is a kind of prison for us, restricting us to our personal desires and to affection for a few persons nearest us. Our tasks must be to free ourselves from the prison by widening our circle of compassion to embrace all living creatures and the whole of nature in its beauty... We shall require a whole new manner of thinking if mankind is to survive.

—Albert Einstein

Five years earlier, I woke dazed and confused from a restless sleep, to the slur of frightening moans. Warm blood stained the fresh paint of the bathroom walls with fierce red splats, crudely signifying the habitual self-abuse my husband suffered. Eight months pregnant, I stood big-bellied, staring in horror at the mutilated body in front of me. From the hallway I faintly heard my three-year-old cheerfully singing, "You are my sunshine." The contrasts in life suddenly were fully lucid.

We all have our ups and downs, our "off" days and our "on" days, but if you're suffering from bipolar disorder, these peaks and valleys are more severe. The dramatic shifts in mood from the highs of mania to the lows of major depression can last for days, weeks, or months. Studies have shown that 25% to 50% of people with bipolar disorder attempt suicide. (CDC, 2005)

Some warning signs of suicide include a change in eating habits, diminished sex interest, change in behavior or personality, and a change in sleeping patterns. A recent loss through divorce, separation, or death can play a big factor in triggering depression and promoting suicidal thoughts. A loss of job, low self-confidence, a diminishing interest in hobbies, and comments of hopelessness are also warning signs.

It is reported that more than half of all suicides occur in adult men ages twenty-five to sixty-five; however, nearly twice as many females attempt suicide. (CDC, 2004)

I fought back the threatening purge of vomit and instead, I jumped into survival mode. I did not understand, because life seemed to be smooth the previous week. It was not until later that I learned that the risk of suicide can be greatest right after the depression lifts. Every eighteen minutes another life is lost to suicide, and this unfortunate alternative to non-acceptance of life takes the lives of nearly thirty thousand Americans every year. (CDC, 2004) But that morning's crisis did not add to those particular statistics.

However, this was not the last time I would face this unfortunate crisis. My perspective was forever changed on the inner battles of the human mind, the effects of choices, and the cycles we grow accustomed to.

The emotional turmoil instigated by the cyclical nature of my former husband's mental illness and the terrifying outbursts of violent rage fragmented what was left of my own sane mind. Tearing at my soul was the unforgiving claws of guilt. I devoutly failed to help my partner. I failed as a wife, and I failed to meet expectations within myself that were proudly set, yet established far beyond reason.

My anger lay eerily dormant, waiting to erupt as it

bubbled internally until my mind melted under the self-created pressures of guilt, fear, and depression. Trapped in the solemn clutches of self-judgment, and fearful of what others would think, I hid from the world and camouflaged my inadequacies. Being near others magnified my own faults and misconceptions. The smallest of tasks, which normally I completed with ease, became a mountainous job that threatened my self-created immutable perfection. I couldn't even shop at fluorescent-illuminated stores due to the overwhelming sensation of an oncoming disaster. Worse yet, there was the fear I might run into an acquaintance who would expect to engage in a logical conversation where I'd be forced to muster a smile. In hopes of eliminating any such event, I took on a new style of living, covering my body with a large, black-hooded coat from which I peered cautiously out into the intimidating world. I did no more than hold on and try to survive.

Survival: Continuing to Live, Outlive, Outlast

Survival is being able to adapt to any living condition — famine, sexual abuse, illness, assault, etc. You must protect yourself; deal with your emotions, fears, and beliefs. Even the act of learning how to make the most out of each day is part of survival. Part of adapting is being able to make choices for you and taking not only an interest in, but also active steps toward, a continuing existence.

In the harsh winter of 1846-47, the unyielding survival rate for the Donner Party crossing over the Sierra Nevada Mountains was slim. Few lived through the bitter cold and famine.

> **Almost invariably, people who come through harrowing experiences are those who believe they can.**

Like the pioneers of the Donner Party, there are courageous people who recognize such a challenge as something to overcome. They may not even consider failure a possibility. The most important characteristic shared by survivors of wilderness emergencies—the will to live—is the same for the abuse survivor, the cancer patient, or the self-destructive person. Successful self-defense occurs when the survival mode is working at its best.

Hopefully you will not need to eat people to stay alive as the Donner Party did; however, when surviving traumatic occurrences, strengthening your spiritual growth, or simply experiencing daily life, it may feel, at times, as if you are being eaten alive by your own haunting self-worth—or gnawed on by those around you. The moment of survival is when you find out who you really are, what you are really made of. When I speak of survival, I mean surviving on whatever path you are on, as an individual and as a member of society. Many of us have the essentials as well as several added luxuries that the pioneers and other historic figures of the past were not concerned about. Fitting in and feeling good about you, while quieting the mind and believing in yourself, comprise another level of survival to strive for. Unfortunately, sometimes when we have many luxuries, there is tendency to become lazy and less appreciative. Our expectations may bring about unrealistic needs and wants, causing blindness to the reality of what is truly important.

What Is Truly Important

When utilizing physical self-defense, it is of utmost importance to keep the mind open, free, and flowing so we can react quickly and instinctively to any confrontation or dangerous situation as it arises.

> *The mind must be emancipated from old habits, prejudices, restrictive thought processes, and even ordinary thought itself...scratch away all the dirt your being has accumulated and reveal reality in its is-ness, or in its such-ness, or in its nakedness.*
> —Bruce Lee

If the martial artist studies the essence of Shinobi, which is a process vital in protecting oneself, and learns its skills, he or she will also gain the secret of Kanjin Kaname: "what is truly important."

So what is truly important? Balance. The principles of nature unconditionally provide flow, harmony, truth, and light, which we also seek for self-protection. Take for example, the five elements: fire, wood, water, metal, and earth. Without earth, no other element could exist. Having no earth within our elements would be like having no truth in light or having no flow in harmony. In the same way, strengthening, supporting, and healing each aspect of the mind, body, and spirit is important. Combined, the mind, body, and spirit provide a balanced foundation from which to perform, both externally and internally. With lack of flow in the physical body, we become rigid, stiff, and move slowly. If there is no flow in the spirit, then we become blocked and limited in a variety of ways that may show up as lack of creativity, trust, faith, or belief. Without the flow of an open mind, we become fixed, static, and remain confined within our own modes of thought.

The result is a lack of harmony and balance that produces a "stuck" feeling or a situation that is difficult to break away from. The tricks of the mind can hold us fixed in a worldview that does not serve us at all if we don't remain open and fluid with change. The ego keeps us attached to past pain, holding us prisoner to the past through our own agreement to listen to the continuous chatter of guilt, shame, and pain. It drains our power, the very voice of our individualism and self-importance.

The Ninja trained the mind, body, and spirit for self-protection, as they were trained to avoid unnecessary conflict and strive to merge their spirit and technique into one. They became known as the "uncommon" common person. Ninjas believed in finding and facing their fears so they could find and live their power. Masaaki Hatsumi, 34th grandmaster of Ninjutsu, offers insight into such training in his book, The Way of the Ninja:

"The ninja would protect himself with techniques not of assassination but rather of sensation and an acute awareness of his natural surroundings. Their harsh training endowed them with a tough but pliant spirit, and martial skills suitable for coping with any situation, together with a sense of awareness and universal application."

Sometimes the Ninja (like natural healers) are viewed as mystical, as wizards or witches, but they are really no different from any of us. They are ordinary people who have developed skills in order to survive difficult times.

Although we may not achieve mental stillness with the same execution as the elite Ninja, we do have the choice to step out of false images and beliefs we have created about ourselves. We can stop creating our self-images with the use of other people's words and our own false judgments. Forget the past; we can dwell for the rest of this lifetime on past lives and old memories. However, in a way, that is simpler. It takes more gumption to let go of the past and start here, now.

Psychosymmetrolysis: The Ninja of the Healing World

You will find many parallels in the training of the Ninja. You will find parallels also in the study of Psychosymmetrolysis (PSY), a method of understanding nature's ability to find its own course of healing. "Psycho" is mind, "symmetry" is perfect balance and equality, and "trolysis" is a process. Psychosymmetrolysis is built upon the most effective theories and methods of natural healing, evolving from healing traditions from over two thousand years ago. PSY focuses on the subtle energies that surround all living things. The approach is simple, the technique is easy to apply, but the process is complex. Activating the art of natural healing compliments and supports a well-rounded self-defense system.

Sometimes the old-fashioned methods still work, and you can't get anymore old-fashioned then natural healing.
—Ondre

From perseverance, patience, and compassion evolves a complete form of self-protection. The four pillars in the activation process of self-healing and promoting self-protection are:

1. The Mind: Gain trust and appreciation of oneself.
2. The Body: Do to your body what you want your body to return to you.
3. The Spirit: Revitalize through experiences with supreme love, having faith in something of higher frequency.
4. Empowerment: The self-acclaimed vigor that manifests from combining the first three pillars and that which is deeply rooted in belief.

Ninja training, as well as many forms of martial arts similar to the natural healing art of PSY, emphasizes mental discipline and the exploration of consciousness and human potential.

Flow: The Quiet Mind in Action

As stated in Pychosymmetrolysis, there is a constant and natural flow in nature that goes unobstructed from one point to the next. For strengthening and protecting the mind, body, and spirit, flow is essential to omit any stagnation or blockages. Let's put it this way: if you are physically, mentally, or spiritually constipated everything is backed up, slowed down, or completely blocked.

On the other hand, if you suffer from physical, mental, or spiritual diarrhea, everything spurts uncontrollably while vital nutrition is depleted and inspiration is lost. There may even be unclear emotions and a lack of sanity. When sparring against a partner in the martial arts, it is essential to have conscious flow in both your physical movements, as speed, precision, and accuracy are important. How to acquire the presence of flow within the emotions is a life-saving technique. When you face someone in a non-threatening sparring session or in a threatening assault situation, you must maintain control at all times. The most aggressive fighter is not necessarily the one in control. Often the aggressive sparring partner advances out of anger or fear. Although anger or fear can help drive the person, the effect can be devastating if nothing positive supports the emotion. Maintaining control does not mean being completely devoid of emotion, rather it is to understand or accept your emotions so that your mind is able to enter a quiet, focused state.

From this centered state, awareness awakens to help detect what move your opponent may throw next and notifies you where his or her weaknesses are. If you have too much control, your awareness and intuition become blocked, but if you allow flow within a controlled mind, this will produce effective results. Sometimes we find ourselves the stuck victims of a trip-up in the mind, a physical confrontation, or spiritual loss. Similar to a sparring/self-defense situation or dealing with relation-ships of all sorts, it takes a simple physical switch of pace, a mentally fresh approach, or an increase of energy to produce more flow and to gain positive control and a renewed vision of the situation. Do not become stagnant! Get out of that corner; make the move, and go for it! Become a predictable unpredictability and stay one step ahead of your opponent; that is the same as being in control of your emotions, while allowing the harmony of flow to provide a launching pad for action.

For example, flow is intensely present in the work of any true artist. I watched my friend begin to paint as she gazed across the aqua waters connecting the tropical Hawaiian Islands. I was awed by her agility in creating a masterpiece of color, story, and emotion. I saw the creativity flow through her in a focused controlled manifestation, yet she was completely improvisational and allowing at the same time.

Creativity and creation are something that all living beings must do and are one in the same. We all start off as a lump of clay, and life, our hopes, and aspirations form us. Then life's lessons fire the clay, and we ourselves do the final decorating.

—Ondre

Because PSY is essentially the process of balancing and harmonizing the entire self, it can be looked upon as an efficient self-protection course with the solid foundation of heightened awareness. Combining PSY self-healing principles and physical self-defense techniques offers a multiple level approach to the potential external and internal dangers we face daily.

These steps can help prevent one from becoming a victim of phony spiritual quests or a victim of crime. Also worthwhile is gaining knowledge and understanding of potential assailants. We are surrounded by crime daily. Whether it is a violent crime inflicted by another or the agony of self-exploitation, if we are attentive, both can be prevented.

**Awareness is prevention—
Prevention is our number one defense.**

Chapter Three

Knowledge is Power:
Awareness of the Assailant

When in despair, I remember that all through history the way of truth and love has always won. There have been tyrants and murderers, and for a time they seem invincible, but in the end they always fall.

—Mahatma Ghandi

The importance of having an understanding of potential assailants is not to instill fear. If you have fear of the "bad people" in the world, it is time to turn fear into power. Knowledge creates awareness, and that power can prevent you from being labeled a pleading victim of inflicted crime.

How do we recognize an assailant, an attacker? Surprisingly, a common response to this question results in the description of a grubby, wild-eyed male wearing black clothes with hanging chains, a studded belt, and tattoos covering each of his extremities. For anyone who remembers Ted Bundy, the famous serial killer in the 1960's, this description is far from correct. An attacker can be male or female, of any race or age. Like Ted Bundy, the attacker may dress professionally in a suit and tie, might be a handsome surfer-dude, your favorite teacher, or maybe your smiling next-door neighbor whose favorite hobby is baking pies. In short, a criminal can look, act, talk, and dress like anyone.

Stalking: The Fastest Growing Crime

Sheri 28: A Contagious Smile

I met this guy through a family friend at a small get-together. He seemed nice, quiet, polite, and he was good looking. He was tall and slender, had clean-cut blonde hair, and a contagious smile. He took a keen interest in me, which at the time boosted my self-esteem. We had a long, intimate talk. Thinking back, he asked far more questions than I asked him, and I openly rattled on. Usually I am shy, but when someone seems to have a genuine interest in my life, hobbies, work, and values, it is hard to resist sharing with a listening ear. It felt great to talk with someone with similar ideas and tastes. I couldn't believe how much we had in common.

We continued the chat for weeks via e-mail, but I was not interested in a relationship at the time, so I never instigated the contact. I made the mistake of giving out my home number, and he began calling as often as twelve times per day. He remained soft-spoken, but it became more uncomfortable as he pushed harder for more personal information. I didn't return his calls, and that's when he started to show up at the hospital where I worked. Night after night for two weeks straight, he waited for me to walk to my car, and he asked me to join him for one drink. He said we could visit like old times. He sent me roses and love notes as though we were in some kind of intimate relationship. I now wondered if maybe I was dealing with someone mentally unstable. It was creepy, but I thought he would just go away if I didn't give him any more attention. But, that made it worse; he became seriously persistent.

I was worried. I changed my telephone number. I

started to walk out to my car with a male co-worker, which aggravated and pissed off the guy even more. He became increasingly aggressive and yelled at me that I was not being faithful. He yelled while telling me he loved me and that he knew I needed him. He said he would be good to me, kind,—and give me what I wanted, if I went home with him. Although he never physically hurt me, I feared for my safety when he threatened to take me while I slept if I didn't join him for one Date.

I felt violated. Suddenly my freedom was ripped from me. I was under surveillance twenty-four hours a day by some delusional guy. It is a frightening feeling to not feel safe in your own home. I felt on guard constantly, which became extremely draining. Soon I was unable to sleep at night. I became an emotional wreck and found it hard to focus on my life.

I filed a restraining order and physically removed myself from the situation by living out of town for six weeks at my mother's. I resumed my normal lifestyle, but it took me many months to trust and share with other men or feel secure again. I often wonder; where is he? Is he still out there? Is he now hooked onto another innocent victim?

Stalking has become one of America's fastest growing crimes, producing more than eight thousand prosecutions each year. (Stephan Kurr, 2002) Stalking consists of a pattern of threats and actions intended to frighten, even terrorize. The victim may be hounded by letters, phone calls, or emails. There may be threats of sexual or physical abuse. It destroys one's sense of self-worth and sense of safety. Stalkers display an obsessive personality and may suffer from paranoia, erotomania, schizophrenia, and/or delusional thinking. Stalkers are often above average in intelligence and smarter than the average person with mental problems. They will not take "no" for an answer and, as their every thought is on the person they are pursuing, they will go to great lengths to obtain information in order to relate to and become closer to their victims. Since stalkers usually suffer from low self-esteem and are often loners, they feel they must have a relationship with the victim in order to experience personal self-worth. Instead of seeing this obsessive infatuation as threatening or intimidating, they see it as a means to gain the person's love.

Like most assailants, stalkers want control over their victims and can become frustrated and dangerously violent when they don't get what they want. Statistically, (Stephan Kurr, 2002) two in every ten women will be stalked in their lifetime, as will one in every forty-five men. It is important to note that a potential suitor, friend, or even an acquaintance could become a stalker. Victims of stalking should never take the situation lightly, no matter who the stalkers are, or how close they have been emotionally.

Sexual Offenders

Sexual predators seek power and control and will use any means to dominate their victims. However, predators are terrified of being found out; therefore, they generally portray the role of a submissive and tender person when they are around others. Predators often display sincere warmth and enthusiastic interest in their victim's job or hobbies. They may have strong social skills, engage in community events, social or work events, and seem to be givers who put themselves out for others.

This is the ultimate setup. Predators often have positions of authority and trust in their families, on their jobs, in their communities, groups, or organizations. We are lulled into a blind trust, reassured by a well-rehearsed façade. Sexual assault is different from many street attacks, as it is a premeditated act that predators often plan well in advance. They can act alone, in pairs or groups, or have a confidant, someone to help plan the attack while remaining undercover. Predators do not care what physical or emotional scars they impose on a victim and, although they may not kill anyone, their victims can be left severely damaged physically, emotionally, and spiritually.

According to the Office of Justice Programs of the United States Department of Justice, (BJS http://www.ojp. usdoj.gov/bjs/cvict.htm, 2005) sex offenders are about four times more likely than non-sex offenders to be arrested for another crime after their discharge from prison—5.3% of sex offenders versus 1.3% of non-sex offenders.

Dina, 19: Sexual Assault
I found out that he had the same hobbies as I did. Like he loved water polo and he was raising money so he could buy a Morgan horse like the one I owned. How interesting, I thought, that we had so much in common. He was really friendly and he said he wouldn't mind giving me a ride home. I was happy for the lift.

We got in his car but instead of going toward my house, he drove me to the empty fairgrounds where he parked in the dark under the trees. He became eerily silent. I was scared and knew I had made a big mistake. I did not know how to get away. He locked the car doors, smiled and started stroking me. I yelled and tried pushing him away but it didn't help, it only seemed to make him more excited. He continued to push himself on me and he sexually assaulted me before he pushed me out the car door and raced away. I was left alone, shaking with terror. Thankfully, I lived, but I felt dead and dirty.

Serial Killers

Definitions of serial killings vary between states, governments, and nations, but the unique element in serial killing that separates it from other types of murder is that the series of killings do not relate to events surrounding one another.

There are three common characteristics found in most serial killers during their childhood. Called the terrible triad, they are:

1) 60% of serial killers wet the bed past twelve years of age;
2) A fascination with arson; and
3) Animal torture.

Although they may present themselves in a decent or charming way in public, their thoughts are far from appropriate. You may have heard of Charles Manson, Ed Gein, Ted Bundy, and Karla Homolka,—just a few notorious serial killers. Despite high IQs, serial killers often do poorly in school or have trouble holding a job. Attacks are triggered by either sexual fantasies or a need to inflict pain and fear. Over seventy-five percent of the world's serial killers hunt for their victims in the United States. Experts believe our culture's acceptance and glorification of violence may be partially to blame. "According to criminologists, at any given time there are at least 25-100 active serial killers in the United States." (ABC World News, 2005) Feeding on the pain and misery of innocent prey, the mind of the psycho can be a fascinating, yet horrifying, reality.

The "Forget Pill"

Heather 23: A Roofie Victim

I remember nothing. I woke feeling bruised, cold, and half naked. I was behind a large dumpster way out behind the bar where I had a few drinks earlier in the evening. I had some casual contacts with a couple of men like I had pursued many times before, but this night was different. My skirt was crudely cut and my shirt torn. I was completely violated, but I had no recollection of the events that hurt me. It was nearly sunrise as I lay there shivering, my mind a blur. I felt scared, confused, and alone.

One of the fastest growing crimes in America is the use of "roofie" or Rohypnol, a silent and devastating date-rape drug. Rohypnol, a sedative that is ten times the strength of Valium, is illegal in the U.S. It dissolves easily in cola, red wine, or any other dark-colored beverage. It is odorless, tasteless, and absorbs rapidly into the body's system. Even limited exposure to the drug will cause confused thinking and impaired judgment as well as nausea and dizziness as you fight to stay conscious. If you have been drugged with this "forget pill," it may cause temporary amnesia, muscle relaxation, sleep, and impaired motor skills. Any trace of the date-rape drug will disappear from your body long before your memory returns. Both women and men are victims of "roofie," with fewer rapes reported by men.

If, even after a couple sips of a drink, you begin to feel dizzy, confused, or nauseous, you may have been drugged. Seek help immediately from someone you can trust.

Ryan, 42: Too Good to Be True

I sat at the table across from this beautiful woman who was a couple years younger than I. I couldn't believe she was my date. She was sexy, ambitious, financially stable, and she had these incredible green eyes—this was too good to be true. I was excited to take her to my favorite local restaurant where I was known to dine alone most evenings. We ordered drinks and I then excused myself to use the restroom. When I returned there was a waitress at the table and she apologetically said, "I'm sorry I got you the wrong drink," and she took away my red wine.

I was unaware when I was in the bathroom, my date slipped a pill into my drink, and the waitress, who just happened to notice this, quickly took my glass, fearing that something was wrong. The waitress took the glass into the back and notified other workers who agreed that they saw a slight white powder in the bottom of the drink.

Later in the evening I went out for a smoke and, apparently, my beautiful date struck again. She slipped a pill into the remainder of my wine and, again, the waitress, who was keeping a close eye, saw this. When I returned, my glass was gone from the table. My date looked a bit disturbed, and I thought it rude that they cleared our drinks so suddenly when I only left for a quick smoke.

I approached the counter to complain about this unnecessary bussing of my table. I was met by the waitress, a waiter, and the manager; all had distraught looks on their faces. Before I could utter a word, they explained that, not only once, but twice, my sexy, financially stable, too-good-to-be-true date had slipped a pill into my drink. They saved the infected glasses of wine in the back. Although the white powder was no longer visible to the eye, I agreed to them calling the police. The police did a test and sure enough, I was almost drugged.

I never thought that would happen to me, not just because I am a man, but because I thought I could discern character better than that. I am more careful now. Unfortunately, that date was too good to be true.

We can be victimized by assault, dominated by others, or victims of our own ignorance.

Chapter 4

Spiritual Pretention

Without knowledge, there is ignorance. Where there is ignorance there is anger, hate, and poor choices.
—Ondre

Lost in a whimsical and dreamy mind, I thought I was now on my way to spiritual mastery. I found a teacher, and I meditated regularly. I consumed an organic vegetarian diet. With a fond craving for baked tofu, I spoke softly and listened diligently to George Winston's peaceful piano tunes. It was irrelevant to me at the time that I forgot to pray, except for the reoccurring times it felt like my life was falling apart. That is when I suddenly became the holy-roller with flailing hand movements and wild voice fluctuations that made even the dog slink out the door to give me extra space. If the praying did not prove immediately helpful, I turned to sweets as a sedative for masking frustrating emotions.

How easy it was, even in the rumbling shame of my gassy stomach, to look down upon people who listened to loud, obnoxious noise they referred to as groovy music, people who drove fancy cars, and those who stuffed their faces with McDonald's burgers, milkshakes, and greasy fries.

In becoming what I thought was spiritual, I instead created a blinded world wherein I felt safe. Anything that threatened my conditioned beliefs or sense of control was immediately deemed negative, a waste of time, or just plain inconceivable. On the outside I appeared calm and collected. Yet inside, the jumble of emotions, confusion, and self-created lies ate at my soul, tearing the very essence of life from me.

A false sense of spirituality makes for a vulnerable time for a new "convert." It is a phase at the beginning of any transformation, when you are open to the world, both the positive and negative, without possessing much of a personal filter. With contrasting views, stemming from old belief patterns and ego conditioning, it is a time that can feel wonderful, scary, exciting, overwhelming, depressing, hopeful, helpless, or all of the above. In short, it can feel like an emotional roller coaster ride through flames of hell, intertwined with uplifting angelic moments.

The Importance of Working on Self

Despite the turmoil and drenched within the egos mischievous nature, I felt pretty good about myself and actually liked myself quite a bit. The more my motor revved, the less I wanted to see what substance still might lie under my hood. Much to my horror, my impaired ego—struck with the weaknesses of expectation, attachment, and fear—was soon revealed, as my newfound teacher was not a magician with a glittering wand. Instead he was some sort of down to earth, spiritual mechanic who had no fear of the complications, grease, or grime that accompanies the drudgery of rebuilding one's belief system.

Honestly, I am not that knowledgeable in the mechanics of a car, but there were those days—they always seemed to be the cold, rainy afternoons—when my dad dragged me to the garage and insisted that I be self-reliant enough to at least change a flat tire. So, there I sat on the freezing concrete, struggling less with the lug nuts, but more with my dramatized, mind-boggled questioning of this seemingly unnecessary experience. We poked our heads under the hood and my father spoke passionately in what, I felt, was some foreign language. He explained various parts of the engine and lectured on how important it is to keep the contents under the hood clean and well-kept so all systems can continue to work properly together. I still don't know much about cars, but I must say I did gain an appreciation for this contraption that transports my family to numerous metro-soccer games, volleyball scrimmages, improvisation acting classes, grocery stores, music lessons, and to and from work. They really are magnificent hunks of metal.

Ondre is a very efficient, effective spiritual mechanic who spends quality time on even the smallest of details whether he is working on a car, with an animal, with plants—a single cell or the entire human being. He can pinpoint the low oil level, locate the miniscule crack in the cylinder and warn you of a loose fan belt with tremendous accuracy and speed. What's more, he can help drain dirty oil and give you five fresh quarts to load, but he won't put it in for you. He may suggest a few options for how to rebuild your spiritual engine, but ultimately, you must get your own hands dirty, take responsiblity and do the job yourself.

"People want everything—now. I have never taught people in America before, so this is a whole new learning curve for me. I realize that people here expect it to be the same as everything else, like school. And you know what? It's not school. People are not as open to change in America as in other countries. Apparently you go to school here and, as long as you do well in school, you get rewarded for it. People want pats on the backs, rewards, and they want to follow structure. Experiential learning is like: here is the situation, fix it. You do problem solving, and people don't usually want that. They want leadership and concise order.

35

I am a person who believes you should do it yourself. Who the hell am I to tell you what to do? So, class is sometimes a mixture of what people want me to tell them and what I believe I really should say. That can be an issue. Also, it is completely frustrating to the student because, at first, it seems like everything is contradictory until they put all the pieces together and it starts to make sense. They don't particularly want to listen to a process or how it's done, so they try to change it to make it work to fit their needs, and then it doesn't work and they wonder why. It takes dedication, it takes desire to do this kind of work."
—Ondre

I was not a religious person, at least not by the defined fashion of those who rate it by church attendance, and I rarely gave prayer a thought unless I was in desperate emotional need. Randomly I prayed, while not giving much credit to those above at first. Oh, the joys of spiritual pretension—spiritual flatulence. See what you want to see. Hear what you want to hear. Eat what you want to eat. Eventually this blissful state caught up with me and demanded that I take responsibility for my life.

But I began to notice that the more I prayed, the more odd occurrences started happening around me. I admit that I respond in breathless excitement at the mention of any paranormal encounters or things otherwise unexplainable.

It was a Tuesday morning when I sat in my car stopped at the stoplight. I noticed a man dressed in green and brown camouflage and a maroon beret. He stood tall on the corner of the sidewalk. He began to walk quickly through the crosswalk, taking long strides right in front of me. I suddenly realized that this man had no feet and no part of him was touching the ground. From three car lengths away (and I was wearing my glasses) I could see that his pants narrowed near the bottom of his legs as if they were tucked into tall combat boots, but he had no feet and no boots—nothing visible to hold him up. His pants ended a foot above the ground. The soldier continued to walk footless and, as soon as he was half way across the crosswalk, he suddenly vanished. I looked all about expecting to see him, but he was gone and other drivers showed no sign of surprise or acknowledgment that they had witnessed the sight of this lone solider.

The supernatural is the natural not yet understood.
—Elbert Hubbard

Without our individual beliefs regarding the presence or lack of presence of the divine, we would live in boring existence. Some people do not believe in God, ghosts, or spirit guides, and it is not for any of us to judge. But I happen to be a firm believer in all of the above. However, it was not until I finally took notice that my prayers were being heard that I gave proper respect and acknowledgment to those "upstairs."

I lived through many years when even the thought of The Universe, The Great Void, The Great Light, The Creator, or whatever manifestation of God's name was mentioned, made me angry or bitter. The Darwin fish swimming on the rear of many cars was my favorite logo, almost to the point of rebellion. Even though I have cried out for help from the great teacher of peace, called Jesus, it was always a bit hard to digest the set ordinance suggesting that Christ is the only path to God, so I have responded to the transcendent mystics of all religions. Skipping the argument about whether or not God exists, and skipping the "box-shattering" view of whether or not spirits exist, I have always responded with earnest excitement to anyone who has ever said that God does not live in a dogmatic scripture or in a remote throne of gold high in the sky, but instead abides very close to us—closer than we may ever imagine, within touching distance of our very own hearts.

But why must so many suffer if there is a God, I wondered? Why is there so much pain, torture, and abuse?

It is more comforting sometimes to put blinders on and numb ourselves from the negativity of the world. For example, there are those who choose not to watch TV news or read the daily newspaper because of the misfortune, hate, pain, and evil that is revealed. Some don't want this in their house or around them because they are far too "spiritual." But is this not denial? Isn't it far better to be aware of how the world is ticking and to know what kind of world we live in?

Many of us are concerned with developing personal growth, but if we shy away from the very truth of what is happening around us, how can we understand what is happening within us?

If you suffer from spiritual flatulence, you are not alone in this cushioned hole. But indeed it may be time to open the mind to what really is out there—both the good and the bad. In some interviews I conducted with Ondre, he explained the world he sees and deals with as an "intuitive" on a daily basis. Although it may not seem like it, interestingly enough, it is the same world that you and I live in.

"People watch horror films and get scared, but what I see in the real world is far worse. All the horrors you see in films

created by people are just fantasy. The reality is far worse. As an intuitive healer and medium, I see the remnants of what people have had done to them. I see everything from men, women, and children who have been raped, people who have been tortured, people who have had their babies taken from them to be used in cult practices, and I have seen young men and women who have had body parts cut off—mostly men, as they get the worst of the torture. They can do some pretty horrific things to each other like using hot iron rods and various implements. Women are not immune to this. There are a lot more films out there that show women being captured, thrown into pits and tortured. Some films breed a culture of people who want to do those things. It is hard to imagine that someone will watch a horror film and want to replicate what they see being done, but there are those who actually get a thrill out of it. And then they want to try it, they want to kill somebody, they want to torture somebody.

It is unfortunate that films perpetuate this, but they are, and they are becoming increasingly more detailed. The film, The Blair Witch Project, where women capture young men and take them to torture, is just a film, but these things are really happening. People go missing daily. Most of the children end up in slavery as prostitutes, or dead.

There is a human desire for murdering children that is not going away, and it is not being dealt with. Pedophilia is very strong in this country as it is around the world. It is worse in Europe where children are murdered, raped, and tortured, while being videoed. I worked with the police for a period of time as we traveled across Europe. I was shown some videos to introduce me to the crime. Bestiality, torture and, ultimately, murder, was what I saw. One young girl, only six, was surrounded by men who beat and tortured her over a period of months and then peeled her skin off until she was dead. That video has made a fortune for those people who made it because, unfortunately, there is a demand from people who want to watch this kind of horror, better known as "snuff" films. The perpetuators of this evil enjoy performing the torture and cruelty, and the viewers enjoy watching it.

If we go back in history and look at what the Romans did to people, what the ancient Greeks—or Hitler—did, today may not be as violent, but the aggression is just as prevalent. It is about power and control. It is all about energy. The perpetrators feel powerful when they take someone's life. Their ultimate power is to take innocence. It is evil, yet people enjoy it.

So, there is a different kind of character. When people say to me that the world is perfect, that there are some bad people out there, but not many, and everybody has a core essence and beauty...they can say that—but from my experiences, there are definitely those who are light and those who are dark. Many healers disagree with me and say that all people are good. Though there are many incredibly good people out there—I found that not to be true in all cases."

I asked Ondre about spirit guides because since childhood I possessed a passion and desire to know more about what is beyond our naked eye and media-addicted world. From the time I was six until about age thirteen, I distinctly remember conversing with someone or something that didn't have a physical presence. To an onlooker it may seem like I had an overly active imagination, and perhaps I did. But I cannot deny that, at those times, which were usually in the isolation of my bedroom or in the comfort of our musty barn, I felt a heightened sense of ease. I felt accepted, content, and understood.

Anything considered within the realms of ghosts, intuition, or the supernatural fascinated me because it offered possibilities beyond the logical mind. The controversy of these misunderstood subjects created a stir if brought up in conversation, and it certainly peaked my curiosity for that which I gladly welcomed, to wake things up in an otherwise seemingly flat worldview.

Through many unexplained occurrences—too many to note here—and in witnessing profound healing during my studies in Psychosymmetrolysis, I acquired a deep-rooted belief in the spiritual world.

> **It can be scary to open up to the possibilities of all that truly surrounds us, but usually it is only scary because it threatens to challenge our preconditioned beliefs or strikes the fear that, believe it or not, we are not in control of everything.**

I share again words from Ondre, and I offer this with the intent to pass along the perspective from a world-renowned professional medium who deals with the spirit world daily. Besides that, Ondre is the most down-to-earth guy I ever met. It may sound like a stewing contradiction but, as noted before, the contradictions in life become more subtle as the mind quiets and expands...

"Everybody has a spirit guide—usually a family member, or someone from a past life, or someone who has had some association with you at some point. Some just pop in because they want to help you. There are good and bad spirit guides and, just like people, some give good advice and some bad. It is kind of like a schoolteacher—you get a good one or a bad one. You get what you get.

If you are a young man or woman who has had a really tough life of abuse or hurt, your spirit guides tend to be strong and powerful. The more you need them, the more they seem to be there. The people who struggle more have stronger spirit guides. On the other hand, people who are spoiled or unthankful tend to have spirit guides who are less powerful. If you do not want to believe in spirit guides, that is fine. People say there is no God, when you die you turn to dust and that is it. Everyone has a personal opinion and, if you do not want to believe that there is someone there to help you, then that's fine. If you do not want to believe in spirit guides, it is purely your choice, but you are missing out on something. Some people used to believe that the world was flat and you could fall off the edge. People who don't believe in spirit guides live in a flat world.

Spirit guides tend to be like you and me, but not in a physical form. They are usually from higher echelons and tend to be attached to a person in order to help the person. A ghost you might see in physical form; spirit guides, you rarely see, but they are always around us. You can have one to one million spirit guides, depending on what help you need, and what you want to achieve. Most people have one spirit guide, and some people are not guided at all because they push the help away. You can't be forced to have a spirit guide, and you can deny the support through drugs, alcohol, or other destructive behaviors. You can recognize those people who do not have spirit guides—they are lost souls.

The spirit world is a lot more forgiving than we are and often even the worst of the worst people still have some guide, trying to help them—sometimes something good and sometimes something bad. I would like to think that if we do good things, good things come back to us. But sometimes the innocent become prey. So, spirit guides are there to try to help prevent that, but even the nicest of people can become victim to the darker side. If you think everything is good and nice, you are in for a real shock."

Abuse, robbery, physical assault, and homicide have become commonplace, so why do the majority of us believe such things will never happen to us?

Even though we see crime on television or read about daily crime in the local newspapers each day, we dismiss the notion that it could be our mutilated body shown on the television screen or our own child's face plastered under the bold typed letters that form the heart-wrenching words: missing child. In our very own neighborhoods we are surrounded by rapists, thieves, stalkers, and drug dealers. It is foolish to assume that one is immune to crime, just as it is foolish to assume one is immune to the personal internal battles of addiction, control, destructive and/or violent behaviors. Sometimes the danger even lives within our own homes.

Chapter Five

The Enemy Within: Domestic Violence

We know what a person thinks—not when he tells us what he thinks, but by his actions.
                    —Isaac Singer

I dedicate two chapters of this book to domestic violence. The need to spread information about the severity and commonality of domestic violence is prompted by the many domestic violence victims I have worked with, as well as the abuse I endured. Perhaps you are suffering from an abusive relationship right now, or maybe you never set foot or heart in this territory. But either way, the effects of domestic violence surround us daily. The complexity of intimate abuse is difficult to recognize, and my hope is to promote prevention that can be used to help you, family members, friends, or your next-door neighbor avoid intimate violence.

According to the Department of Justice report on the National Violence Against Women Survey (November, 2006), each year more than one and one half million women, and three-quarters of a million men, are victims of physical violence by someone they know intimately. That means that "every 37.8 seconds, somewhere in America, a man is battered. Every 20.9 seconds, somewhere in America, a woman is battered."(http://www.men.org/battered/gjdvdata.htm)

Domestic violence is a pattern of behavior used by an individual to establish and maintain control over his/her intimate partner. Unfortunately, it is a common yet often misinterpreted or overlooked problem that occurs within our homes, our communities, and throughout our world.

Domestic violence consists of physical, sexual, psychological, and/or emotional abuse.

Physical signs of abuse include, but are not limited to:

- Pushing, shoving
- Refusal to meet physical needs of dependents
- Choking, beating, shaking, bruising
- Withholding sex and/or affection
- Hitting, punching, kicking
- Throwing victim
- Abuse during pregnancy
- Use of weapons
- Murder

Sexual signs of abuse include, but are not limited to:

- Sexual jokes or demeaning gender-related remarks
- Jealousy, assuming or accusing you of being, or wanting to be, with others sexually
- Unwanted touching, criticism of sexuality
- Name calling with sexual epithets
- Forced to look at or engage in pornography
- Forced sex (rape)
- Forceful, uncomfortable sex
- Rape resulting in permanent injury

In a 2005-06 study conducted in the fifty states and the District of Columbia—based on a survey of sixteen thousand participants, equally male and female—nearly

25% of women and 7.6% of men were raped and/or physically assaulted by a current or former spouse, cohabitating partner, or dating partner/acquaintance at some time in their lifetime.

Psychological signs of abuse include, but are not limited to:
- Jokes and insults
- Ignoring or minimizing feelings
- Yelling, name calling
- Belittling and private or public humiliation
- Blaming and accusing
- Abuser demanding all the attention
- Resentment of marriage and children
- Providing mixed signals
- Lack of cause and effect
- Depression, nervous breakdown
- Mental illness
- Complete isolation and withdrawal

Emotional/social signs of abuse include, but are not limited to the following:

- Uses gender myths and roles
- Degrades culture, religion, nationality, profession, or gender
- Destroys or damages victim's property
- Demonstrates strength
- Controls major finances
- Denies victim's ability to work
- Threatens to hurt victim's extended family or pets
- Eliminates support system
- Keeps the victim in complete isolation
- Commits child abuse/incest
- Alienates victim's family and friends

- Creates victims
- Convinces victims that they are the unstable ones

Although men are more likely to be victims of violent crime overall, a 2003 study by the U. S. Department of Justice reported that "intimate violence is primarily a crime against women." Of those victimized, eighty-five percent are women and fifteen percent are men. It is estimated that only half of all domestic violence incidents are reported to the police. This is common because many victims either view the matter as private, fear retaliation from their abuser, or they don't believe the police can do anything about it.

Although it is said that domestic violence is primarily a crime against women, it is possible that the low percentage of reported violence against men has to do with the disbelief that men could be victims of domestic abuse and violence, and that many men will not even attempt to report the situation.

Jan Dimmitt, executive director of Kelso, an emergency support shelter in Washington that provides free services, education, safety, and support to victims and survivors of domestic/sexual violence, explains, "Whenever I speak of male abuse, I am met with disbelief and, even worse, laughter. We are looked upon as being the friends of the perpetrators rather than friends of the victims, because all males are supposed to be evil and bad. I notice in talking with other shelter staff throughout the state that this attitude prevails in the other shelters, too—that men are the perpetrators, women are the victims."

The impact of domestic violence is less apparent and less likely to come to the attention of others when men are abused. For example, if a man is seen with a black eye, it is automatically assumed that he has been in a fight with another man, bruised by a contact sport or hurt on the job. There have been few resources that address and understand the issues of domestic abuse and violence against men.

In one case, a man was out drinking and came home to fall asleep on the couch. His wife took an iron skillet and beat him. He was taken to the emergency room of the hospital and stitched up. Although it was the police who witnessed the mess and transported him to the hospital, no charges were filed against his wife. My heart goes out to the men who call for help because few services are available to them, other than a psychologist or psychiatrist. I feel we are still in the Dark Ages with our stereotypically view of males and domestic abuse.

According to Philip Cook, whose book, *Abused Men: The Hidden Side of Violence*, tells the above story, Kelso and the Valley Oasis Shelter program in Lancaster, California, and "a few other places" are the only programs in the United States that serve men. Domestic abuse against men and women have similarities and differences. The above-listed aspects of physical violence may be the same for both sexes. However, what hurts a man mentally and emotionally may be very different from what hurts a woman.

Unkind and cruel words can hurt, but they can hurt and linger in different ways. Some professionals have observed that mental and emotional abuse can be an area where women are often more brutal than men. In most cases, men are more deeply affected by emotional abuse than physical abuse. Men and women stay in abusive relationships for similar reasons. Some assume blame if they are guilt-prone. A man may believe something is his fault or feel he deserves the treatment he receives. Other reasons for staying include: to protect his children, fear that he may never get to see the children again, or fear that the woman will tell their children that he is a bad person. The idea of leaving the relationship can also produce feelings of depression and anxiety. In a twisted way, it's as if the partners in the couple become addicted to each other.

Bill, 33: Defining Loneliness

Four years into our thirteen-year marriage, she started becoming cold and angry. She blamed things on me like why we didn't have any extra money and why our life was hard. She told me that she didn't need a man in her life and I was holding her back from being happier and more successful. She told me I was in better shape a few years ago. She pulled out pictures of me when friends came over and showed them how I used to look, even though I was still in good shape at the time. She constantly told me that I was controlling, a jerk, and she made me feel very bad about myself in general. She withheld sex or any form of intimacy. Our relationship was a roller-coaster ride—one or the other of us wanting to get divorced. Then we would pull each other back at the brink in the last moment.

I often wondered why I was staying with her. In my youth, having come from parents who were divorced, I made a commitment to myself, and my wife, that I would never get a divorce. Knowing this, she knew she could take advantage of me because I was not going to leave.

One morning at about 3 a.m., while I watched TV (she did not want me in bed with her), a famous singer was being interviewed. The last question of the interview, the host asked, "Oh, by the way, I heard you are getting divorced again. Isn't this your eighth marriage? Won't you be lonely?" The singer looked shocked for a moment to be asked such a question on national TV. Then I saw her relax and say, "You're right, I have been married eight times and I just seem to make bad choices, but I'm not lonely. Loneliness is being in a bad relationship."

At that moment I realized I could no longer tolerate such loneliness in my life. That night it felt like a flower inside of my chest finally finished withering and, like a dead leaf in the fall, it fell away from me. Although I still felt compassion for my wife, the love, affection, and tender feelings were gone forever. I announced this to her the next morning. Shortly after our separation every part of my life improved. Out of compassion I tried to help her still, but realized I could not.

One example that sticks out was when she called crying one stormy winter morning and said her tire was flat, she was going to be late for work, and she couldn't turn the lug nuts. I went over in the cold, crawled in the mud under her truck and repaired the tire. She jumped in the truck without a word of thanks and left me cold, soaking wet, and feeling empty, used, and taken advantage of. That afternoon a friend of mine who worked with my ex called and let me know that she was saying a lot of mean and spiteful things about me.

Stunned, I said, "Today she said these things?"

Her reply was "Yes, just moments ago, I just thought you should be aware of it."

That night I confronted my ex with her hurtful behavior and told her I would never do anything for her again. I told her that even if I saw her broken down on the road, I would drive by her. That day I broke the cycle of being abused, disrespected, and just plain being treated badly.

I noticed a connection between my breaking this

cycle and something I learned while involved in one of my favorite pastimes. I have made a point of talking with old, grumpy people. It started out as fun, but then I realized, I did not want to become one myself. In my years of impromptu grocery checkout interviews with these crotchety people, I found out they had something in common.

- They spent their life living in a place they did not want to be: for example, they lived in the mountains when they yearned to live at sea.
- They did a job that they hated for thirty to forty years: for example, a man working in sales when his true desire was to build boats.
- They lived with someone for most of their life who they couldn't stand.

On many occasions, the grumpiest of people had experienced all three. I looked at my life and I loved where I lived, I loved my profession, and I now loved myself as a single person... I decided it was much better to be by myself and to be happy than to be lonely and in a bad relationship.

Abusive women are notorious for nagging and criticizing. They often want to change their partner to fit their idea of how their man should be, while having unrealistic expectations and demands. These women typically experience cycles of anxiety, depression, frustration, and irritability, which they attribute to a man's behavior. There are also certain psychological disorders—ex. borderline personality disorder —in which women may be abusive and violent toward men. The disorder is also associated with suicidal behavior, sexual problems, lying, severe mood swings, and alcohol abuse. They blame men for their personal problems, rather than taking responsibility for their own lives. When men cannot make them feel better, they often assume that the man is trying to make them feel miserable on purpose. Abusive women use sex as a cat-and-mouse game of control and power. And let's not forget jealousy. A woman scorned or a jealous woman is worse than a nest of angry yellow jackets. For no apparent reason, abusive women often attack other women, usually verbally. A woman may feel threatened that another woman is younger or more attractive, whether or not the woman is flirtatious toward the first woman's partner.

Men are good at making excuses, too, but a woman has a knack for coming up with excuses while easily blaming unhappiness on the weather, the box of chocolates she just devoured or, although a serious problem for some, good old PMS is sometimes an overused excuse.

For example, I find it preposterous that my husband throws his dirty clothes toward the laundry basket, which misses and lands two feet away. Why can't he take one step closer and put them in the basket? He states that they end up in the washing machine anyway, so why bother? This drives me batty. My silly habit is to cut my fingernails wherever I happen to be sitting. I don't bother to pick them up because I know I will vacuum soon. This drives my husband batty. These may seem petty examples, but the little annoyances are fuel for a fire.

So, before you deem yourself abusive and begin to fret, know that all of us, men and women, at some point in our lives, criticize, nag or make excuses. My partner and I have since communicated our disapproval of each other's lazy behavior and lack of self-discipline. We both chose to work at improving.

If you are involved in an abusive relationship, communication is usually poor and little or no compromises are made to resolve the issue. Even arguing can be part of a healthy relationship; it is the severity, consistency, and intensity of behavior that make it abusive. Male and female abusers are good at manipulating a situation and justifying their behavior so their victims begin to believe that they are the ones in the wrong.

Jan, 58: Living "Out There"

I did not know I was so vulnerable. When we first met it was due to a spiritual component, or so we thought. We enjoyed hikes together and I especially liked his personality. He had a different character than what I was accustomed to. He was more assertive and upfront than I was, and I liked that about him. He was definitely the initiator, but I happily agreed with the movement forward in our relationship.

After knowing each other for one and a half years, we married and wanted to have children right away. Nine months later we had a baby girl. After that—over several years—we stopped having sex or even making out other than to conceive our other three children. Soon after marriage, I barely saw my husband, for he was gone before the children and I woke, and he returned home after ten at night. I loved being a mother, and I loved my children. I was twenty-seven years old and still had an idealistic outlook on life. I was a little bit "out there." We lived in a community setting and my routine consisted of joining in morning meditation, cooking, harvesting, cleaning, and raising the children.

When we moved to Nevada, I realized it was not just in my marriage that I felt alone. In the high desert, it is amazing how quiet it becomes, and how isolated I felt. The downward spiral began as Todd began to gamble and lost a lot of money. He became more and more hostile as his drinking steadily increased, and the harassment he inflicted upon me came as a complete shock. He was the one spending money, but he came home in the evenings and, while I prepared dinner, he demanded that I tell him how much money I spent that day and where it was spent.

The harassment escalated and the brunt of his frustrations ended up being dumped on my eldest son, usually in a physical fight. I did not understand this irrational behavior. Holes in the walls were punched in order to make a point, and the severe kicks to our two dogs were thrown in fits of anger. I couldn't believe the man I loved could be so hateful, but I was not really scared at this point; it was just unthinkable that it was actually happening in my home.

It was not until he bought a shotgun and threatened to kill himself—and then threatened to kill me, and the children,—that I was scared. I was petrified. I didn't know what to do, where to find help, or whether there was help available. I stayed in the relationship because I was financially dependent—he had the financial control. I didn't even know that I could work while raising kids. If I worked, I wouldn't be able to attend their school functions or be a classroom mom. If I worked, I thought I wouldn't have the energy to make dinner and tuck them into bed. After twenty-six years of living in a verbally, emotionally, and psychologically abusive relationship, I finally knew it was time to leave.

I asked Jan several questions, and here is how she responded.

What have you learned from this experience?

It is important to learn about yourself and about relationships. If something doesn't feel right, know that you have the ability to say "see you later" and get out. After being isolated for so long, friends are especially important. I try to nurture friendships, both male and female. It took me a long time to stand up, feel assertive and know that who I am is just as important as anyone else. I still feel insecurities, but I work through them.

What helped you feel better about yourself?

I took a job at Peaceful Families (an organization that provides services to individuals and families who experience sexual assault and/or family violence, offering interventions, education, and prevention services to the community), and I felt appreciated for the very first time. I felt passionate about this job and the children we helped. I experienced some level of success. I still would like to find a balance between being overly aggressive (I can be pretty competitive) and under-assertive. I'm starting to feel a balance and it feels good.

What advice do you have for others in a similar situation?

Keep going for your education and toward the dreams you live for. Don't feel foolish about asking for help. Stay in touch with friends and family—they can be a good support.

Remember that domestic violence is not always physical abuse; it is not all about hitting, killing, or dragging a body around. It can be manipulatively subtle and still be demoralizing.

Chapter Six

Understanding the Cycle of Abuse

Peace cannot be kept by force. It can only be achieved by understanding.

—Albert Einstein

Why do people continue to hurt themselves through drugs, smoking, food, alcohol, or abusive relationships? It is difficult for the family or friend who witnesses the abuse of a loved one. You may want to shout, "Just get out, pack up and go!" It sounds simple, but can you tell a smoker to stop smoking and expect him to quit that day? Will someone with an eating disorder suddenly eat healthy if you warn: "You may die next week if you don't stop vomiting." Why do people put themselves in harm's way? To hurt or to have pain inflicted on them is part of the self-abuse cycle that the person becomes accustomed to. This can stem from childhood abuse, anger at a previous boyfriend/girlfriend, or a past life. It is what they know; it is their comfort level. Take, for example, those who are magnets to drama crises; as much as they say they want to get away from drama, there they are—eating, breathing, and living it. This is the same for those who put themselves in harm's way. It is not always a fully conscious decision, but it's a choice, which stems from familiarity. This cycle of abuse, self or inflicted upon, becomes a part of an ongoing life of misery and neglect.

In order to recognize the cycle of domestic abuse, we have to know how it looks and what to look for. What is it? What are its stages?

The Cycle of Violence

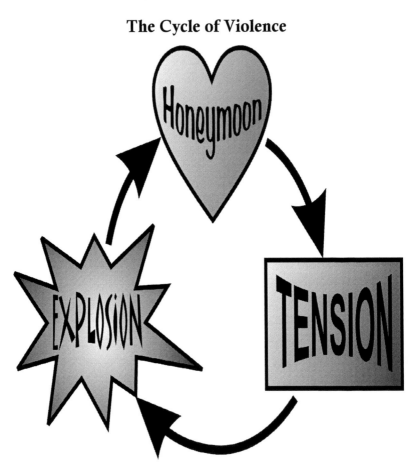

The more times the cycle is repeated, the harder it is to break. In the tension phase you may feel like you're walking on eggshells and experience the need to cooperate with your controlling partner to avoid setting him/her off. The abusive partner is edgy, or moody and unpredictable. By going along with the controlling partner, a victim may feel a sense of false control. This phase may go on for weeks—or months.

The explosion is the most violent and abusive phase, as it is usually concentrated and intense; however, it is often the shortest in length. This phase can be physically or emotionally abusive. Although in an unhealthy way, you "bond" while going through this violence together.

After the explosion, there is the "honeymoon" phase, where there is often love and romance, and you begin to do fun things together. It is this that the victim will miss if the couple breaks up. It is the phase that keeps you hooked into this vicious cycle of violence. A victim can start to feel crazy and not believe he or she was ever scared of his/her partner. The abuser is nice now, creating much confusion and self-doubt in the victim. The victim wants to believe the promise that it won't happen again.

Why Does the Victim Stay?

Personally, I asked myself this question often after five years of living in an abusive relationship. But before answering this question, I came up with every excuse I could to stay in this unhealthy relationship. I did not trust or listen to the feelings that told me to get out. And before that, I did not even recognize that I was in an abusive relationship. It started with small, short temper tantrums and climaxed into bursts of explosive rage. The emotional attacks were so cunningly conceived that I soon felt bad about myself, and lost belief and value in myself as an individual. Becoming isolated and feeling alone, I believed it was my responsibility to fix and care for this person.

The underlying principle in this situation, and for all self-defense, is awareness.

- You cannot accomplish anything without first being aware of your feelings and actions. However, it does not stop there.
- The second part is actually more difficult. You must trust and listen to what you are feeling.
- The third phase is to combine the first two and to act with awareness on those feelings you now trust. It is time to believe in you, and also believe that you can and will safely get out of this abusive relationship.

I thought I was doing a noble deed by accepting the responsibility of my partner's rage. But I wonder, did I also become victim to my own ego as I disregarded my intuition and boldly chanted: "I am strong, I can fix anything, I am strong?"

I did genuinely care for this person, but my fault was that I cared for him more than I cared for myself.

I thought I could help him. Let me tell you, ignorance really is bliss, but very short-lived. As with many victims of domestic abuse, I looked upon divorce as a negative, weak act, and I desperately wanted my children to have a father. The friends and family around me did not see what was happening. My partner was quiet, well mannered, and respected by much of the community. Later, those close to me admitted that they felt something was not quite right about our relationship, but they couldn't place their finger on what was sensed.

Other common reasons victims stay with an abusive partner are:

- They may have lived in a home where abuse was accepted as normal
- The battering may occur over a short period of time and the abuser may convince the victim that this is the last time it will ever happen
- The victim may be economically dependent on the abuser and see no other alternative
- The victim may see no real way to protect herself/himself from the abuser
- The victim may be afraid that, if the crime is reported, the abuser may lose his/her job, which is often the only source of income for the family
- The victim may have no idea of services that are available and feel trapped
- The victim believes she/he has no power to change her/his situation
- The victim is afraid for the safety of any pets left behind (since most battered women's shelters are unable to accept pets).

It is not uncommon for a victim to leave, only to return to the abuser. On the average, the victim leaves and returns seven times before leaving for good. The victim is trapped in this cycle of feeling isolated, helpless, and scared. As the violence escalates in intensity and frequency, the time between phases grows shorter and shorter. However, each victim's circumstances may be different and not fit neatly into this model.

All ages are susceptible to domestic violence. These days, teenage dating violence is on the rise. In fact, "women age sixteen to twenty-four experience the highest per capita rate of intimate partner violence." (http://www.feminist.org/othr/dv/dvfact.html) Are we passing on enough valuable information to our younger generation?

Do we understand it enough to be able to sit down with our daughters and sons and express the dangers and signs of domestic violence? Take the time to learn more about this type of abuse for your sake and for your children.

Sometimes it just takes someone to recognize the signs or to lend an ear to help someone avoid or escape from domestic abuse.

A few years back, I was at the beautiful Yuba River with my family, taking a dip in the refreshing aqua-tinted water, when we were suddenly interrupted by angry shouts and violent splashing. Up river we witnessed what at first looked like harmless teenage play in the middle of the river, but soon we realized it was not so friendly. A young man of about eighteen was holding his hand on top of his girlfriend's head. She looked about sixteen. The boy continued to force her entire body under the water. At first he held her for a few seconds, the next time for many seconds, and the third time for what seemed much too long. She emerged from the water gasping for air, crying and yelling profusely at the same time. The young man shrugged his shoulders. With a confident sneer, and an arrogant twitch of his head, he turned his bulky body and strutted upstream. Before we knew what transpired, the girl suddenly dunked the boy with all her might, returning the agony. When the boy rose from the water, he looked like a wet, ferocious dragon. I almost saw smoke flaring from his nostrils, and the most repulsive and derogatory remarks were fired at her. He raised his hands ready to strike her face, but after noticing us not far from the scene, he changed his mind, cursed her violently and stomped upstream.

The sad part is that the girl, who had just been abused moments before, immediately followed her boyfriend while pleading with him to please forgive her as she excessively apologized for dunking him. His only comments were a loud slur of offensive remarks as he headed upstream toward some of his buddies. I noticed that sitting on the small sandy beach close by were what appeared to be the girl's parents, watching in silence.

What we grow up with becomes our belief and ultimately our reality. The good news is that with hard work, faith, and perseverance, you can overcome this reality and create something new for yourself.

> **It is important to reach out for help.**
> **Know you are not alone.**

If you witness a violent domestic battle, it is usually best to stay out of it. Don't try to be the hero. Many times when you think you may be helping someone, both parties can turn against you. In breaking up a domestic dispute, you might suddenly find yourself the victim. It is safer to report it to the local police station and let them take the matter into their hands.

If you are currently living in an abusive relationship and are ready to get out, you need a simple plan of action:

- Document all abusive behavior that you can in a journal—something that may be used in court. This journal can be kept hidden—at work, a friend's home, anywhere safe. It will be valuable for prosecution, if this need arises.

- Have a bag packed and ready with any important papers, birth certificates, driver's license, as well as clothing for you and your children. This should be ready to go so that, when you decide to leave, you will not have to return.
- Before leaving, make a plan for where you are going to stay that will be safe. The Domestic Violence and Sexual Assault coalition in your community often has safe houses to offer during times of transition.

When you leave, walk out that door proud and strong, knowing that you deserve much better. Don't look back.

Chapter Seven

How Far Do We Go?

Patience is the companion of wisdom.
—Saint Augustine

To fully utilize the mechanics of self-defense, it is important to have some understanding of self, which often means breaking down and rebuilding your foundation—which may be worn, weak, or fractured. This is the beginning point in the healing process of Psychosymmetrolysis, as well as a crucial component for concious self-defense. Get to know yourself. If we do not know our own minds, our selves, and our essence—and those around us do not know who they are—then the entire world we occupy is based on illusion, fantasy, and fear of judgment. Men are sometimes taught to maneuver from their heads and bodies, while ignoring their emotions and spirituality. Women are often taught to be emotional, even spiritual, but ashamed of their intellect and bodies. To succeed in either an assaultive situation, a day on the job, as a parent figure, on a spiritual quest, or in an intimate relationship, you must first know who you are, trust your abilities and care for yourself.

Getting the Right Help

Our culture has become more and more dependent on popping pills to alleviate our headaches, surgery to suck out the overproduced toxic fat, and medication to balance the mind. We don't stop to consider that maybe dehydration caused the headache, a few less French fries and more exercise could remedy the toxic buildup, and maybe a change in pace might ease the mind. Western medicine can be helpful and definitely has its positive sides if used wisely and for certain ailments, however, with the easy and immediate results that medicine can provide, no wonder it is so widely used—and abused. I am both awed by the power of medication and concerned by its prevalence. Medicating the symptom of an illness without finding the core essence of the problem or situation is a backwards way of approaching poor health.

What are we really promoting when magazine ads or television commercials suggest quick relief by consuming medication? If you take this pill, we are practically guaranteed a happier day—or try this one for a better night's sleep. Is media suggesting that there's no need to be responsible for our actions toward our mind and... body? Because—whether we consume alcohol or drugs, have an acid-filled stomach, eat a poor diet, or have an achy muscle—these medications can fix us?

How many people have become reliant on medication to allow them to survive and be a part of each day?

When we pop pills to mask our pain, we are not listening to what our bodies are telling us. An ache or a pain can quite often be a natural warning flag, built into our body to alert us to any imbalance so proper action can take place to re-establish that balance and eliminate the chance of disease. Popping medication merely covers the pain.

It is easy to avoid or forget the use of simple prevention techniques that have the ability to strengthen our wellbeing. For example, flossing teeth is proven to reduce cavities, but not everyone flosses. Learning physical self-defense techniques or CPR can possibly save a life. Checking car tires once a month is recommended to avoid a blowout. Eating oatmeal helps reduce cholesterol. Wearing sunscreen helps prevent skin cancer. There are many simple prevention tools known today that our ancestors either were not fortunate enough to know about or they instinctively used as a means of survival.

Our culture has become dependent on immediate results and there is a lost sense of responsibility for self. Is prevention being pushed aside while numerous "cures" or "fixes" for ailments grab our attention? The wants and needs of immediate gratification are on the rise. This new level of expectation that, unfortunately, today's youths are growing up with, promotes a false sense of healing and survival through medication use, processed foods, and even slathering praise.

The Negative of Positive Praise

Does praise motivate? Sure. It motivates kids, and adults alike,—to get more praise. If you go to the park, a sports game, or even at school, there is one phrase you can count on hearing: "Good job!" As this phrase can be beneficial in supporting and encouraging a youngster, it can also prove to set up a child to be defined by your evaluations or judgments rather than by their personal value within themselves. The reason praise can work in the short run is because often we are hungry for approval.

Contradictory to the assumed reassurance that is given to a child by stating "good job," it ultimately makes them feel less secure.

**Apart from the issue of dependence,
a child deserves to feel pride in personal
accomplishments and also deserves to decide
when that feeling has been earned.**

Each time we say "good job" we are actually telling children how to feel. They instead begin to rely heavily on this given praise to feel that they have succeeded or did well, and this becomes a cycle that encourages children to look outside for acceptance rather than having it come from inner confidence.

There are notable times when it is helpful to say "good job," but the constant flow of positive reinforcement has become almost a verbal tic. For example, we praise someone if they made three soccer goals by saying "good job," and we praise someone who sat on the bench during the entire game by stating "good job." "Good job" is just as much an evaluation as "bad job" and, however you look at it, it is a judgment. And who likes being judged? Instead of diluting your children's enthusiasm for their accomplishment by saying "good job," let them exclaim to you, "I did it!" As a mother I can attest that it is heart wrenching at times when holding back from overly positive remarks on the accomplishments pursued by my children, but what better gift is there than seeing your child flourish in self-approval. It may feel cruel to be kind at times, but in the end it pays off.

It's really less about the number of times we evaluate a "good job," and it is more about the shortcuts that we take as adults to manipulate kids with rewards instead of taking the valuable time to explain and help them develop needed skills and self-respect. Even into adulthood, people may rely on others to "pat them on the back" or tell them that they did well. If this praise is not come by easily, the adult may feel worthless, stupid, carry low confidence in personal ideas and efforts or suffer from low self-esteem.

If you were raised in the midst of gooey slathered praise, beware; or rather be aware, of your reactions when your boss, partner, teacher, or friend does not give you that desired approval. It can be self-destructive and create a great excuse to give up or quit, but actually it is a grand opportunity for growth. The good news is that you don't have to be evaluated in order to succeed. Believe in yourself; listen to your inner strength and wisdom.

Is Natural Beautiful?

I accompanied Ondre on a road trip to Reno, Nevada, where he was scheduled to be a guest on a local radio station. With naïve excitement, I had no idea that we would be met by two radio hosts who would question Ondre in degrading disbelief, and crack jokes on air about his "so-called" healing and "crazy" psychic abilities. Afterwards when we were off the air, Ondre worked on one of the host's injured back and, by the look of pure shock that rapidly spread across this man's wide eyed expression, I could see that some healing took place—on many levels. Ondre seemed unfazed by the previous ridicule, and he now had his mind on the next destination. We went to a hospital, where a caller from the radio show had spoken of his sick mother. We had an hour before the evening's healing forum. Though I would have found comfort in using this limited time to prepare for the forum, Ondre selflessly saw it as the opportunity to assist someone in need.

Upon arriving at the intensive care unit, we were met by Michael, who immediately hugged Ondre as though they were friends of many years. With flowing tears and a raspy voice he told us that his mother had cosmetic surgery. The surgeon reported, after a complication, that Michael's mother had a poor chance of survival due to the high rate of bacteria that had invaded her body.

I never had the slim model's body like the ones I dreamed of resembling in my teenage years. No matter how little I ate, how much I exercised, how hard I tried to squeeze into a size smaller jeans, it took a lot of delusional years before realizing that my broad shoulders and ample hips help me excel in the sports world, but I would never be that size two. What I witnessed that day made me more thankful for the healthy body I do have and encouraged me to be more responsible for its ongoing health.

Michael's mother lay unconscious on the white hospital bed with various machines monitoring her condition. I stood in the corner with my head lowered. I was uncomfortable viewing something so personal. Suddenly the entire room turned stark cold. I jerked my head up with surprise and saw Ondre leaning over the woman's bed deep in prayer. Her body twitched, slightly at first, and then her right hand lifted above her head before it rested on the bed again. Ondre now held her hand, and shivers ran through my body as I witnessed, with the help of the hospital monitors, a miraculous change. The once feeble thump of her heart now matched the rhythm of a vibrant and healthy heartbeat. The clammy ash color of her face turned to a baby pink, and the numbers on the monitors rose steadily. Although I didn't have the knowledge of what these numbers meant, I could tell by the nurses' smiles and inhaled gasps that the change was definitely a positive recovery. At last Ondre whispered to Michael, "That is as far as I can help her. It is now up to your mother if she would like to live or not." Michael nodded without speaking.

Afterwards I asked Ondre why he didn't complete the healing for Michael's mom when I knew he was exceedingly capable and had the unusual ability to do so. As we walked through the intensive care unit he replied quietly:

"It is not about me. Healing in all its forms should always be a choice. Just because someone is restricted to bed, unconscious or in a coma, it doesn't mean to say that the person's spirit is dead. My job is to open the door. However, I am not in control of who comes through it, and the individual makes a choice to accept help or not. All I know is that there is a good door and a bad door—and I open the good door. For some reason I am able to do this.

People upstairs have given me this great gift—sometimes I appreciate it and sometimes it feels like a curse. Some people don't get any benefits from the healing, and other people get miraculous results, but it's not my choice. People have to die, people have to go through difficulties, and people have to get raped and murdered. This is a part of life. It is a terrible process and at some points I can make changes, but I can't fix everything. Can you imagine if no one got sick? We already have a population problem and it would get worse. That is the reason diseases are beating medicine because diseases have to help control the population.

Healing is always a choice. Maybe you want to die and don't want to live any longer. Maybe you are happy the way you are, or maybe destiny says you can't live any longer. I can't make the choice. I can't play God. I am a facilitator. As a healer, I am just part of the process."

That day opened my eyes further into the healing world of Psychosymmetrolysis, the importance of accepting and taking care of one's self, and the ongoing process of self-protection.

We can fall prey, not only to unfortunate crimes, but to the rise of temptations that promise wrinkle-free results, fat reduction, or anti-aging magic. Concious self-defense for the mind, body, and spirit is truly a self-healing process. It is full of choices, speckled with deceptive enticements, stroked by undeniable passions and naughty addictions. But the key aspects to an authentic makeover manifests as inner belief, faith, and the quiet mind.

The only devils in the world are those running around in our own hearts. That is where the battle must be fought.
—Mahatma Gandhi

Chapter Eight

The Mind: Credible or Crazy?

Only in quiet waters do things mirror themselves undistorted.
Only in a quiet mind is adequate perception of the world.
—Hans Margolius

The Truth—A Matter of Perspective

Preservation of the mind begins by breaking down the conditioned truths learned throughout childhood and adolescence—the truths that become ingrained and subtly unquestioned as the correct way of living. The truth you know as your reality. As soon as you step out of the "safe box" you created for your life, you can truly begin to see that which surrounds you. It can be scary to venture from the safety box because suddenly you realize that your truths, and even your morals and values, are merely one person's perception within an ocean of infinity.

A middle school counselor who attended a Safety Awareness Training workshop raised her hand half way through the class looking quite concerned. She asked, "Are we learning these defenses with the thought in our minds that we could be killed if attacked?" I thought for a moment this was a joke, but she was far more serious than a youngster eating a delicately balanced double-sized ice cream cone. She openly admitted that the thought never crossed her mind that another human being could possibly hurt or kill her.

Another lady who was in her late forties told me that she didn't need a self-defense class because she did not participate in any activities that would put her in harm's way. In response to my immediate questions, she commented that her favorite activity is to take nature walks in the wooded trails that run along the river. She liked this because she could be alone, unwind and relax. I found this interesting and contradictory because I had read, only three weeks earlier, that a woman was stabbed on that same trail. The lady I spoke to saw the nature trail in her truth to be a naturally beautiful and serene environment, which in most circumstances it is. However, in her truth, she failed to see that another person's truth (the potential attacker) saw this secluded trail as a golden opportunity to ambush a potential rape victim.

This does not mean to say she must live in fear and no longer take tranquil walks along the wooded river path. But to have an awareness of other perspectives and truths can help prevent a life-threatening situation, or simplify numerous challenges in your daily life.

Do you know anyone who "pushes your buttons" and provides a challenge to see things differently? It can be a boss at work or an employee. Children and spouses can and most certainly will challenge your truth at some point.

For example, my husband thinks everything should be brown in the house—brown couches, brown chairs, brown paint, brown rug—while I think it should be colorful with greens, purples, and maroons.

With unforgiving truth, I believed we needed to attend every field trip with our children's school to be "good" parents. My husband believed we should not attend any so the children could learn independence and gain confidence. Who is right and who is wrong? Neither. It is merely two perceptions of truth.

As you most likely have experienced, relationships can be sticky. This is often due to the endless creations of truth that each individual grows accustomed to through childhood, past lives, previous relationships, illnesses, traumatic experiences, or the need to feel in control. My husband and I finally compromised after numerous squabbles, and we do have a brown house and brown furniture; but some rooms are decorated with uplifting colors. As far as the field trips are concerned, we met somewhere in the middle of our truths, and we attend half during the year.

Another vivid example is a person who suffers from anorexia. His or her truth when looking in the mirror is that of an ugly, gigantic mass of fat, when in reality he or she is starved and barely living. Or, how about someone who suffers from depression? A sunny day on the beach of Hawaii's North Shore can rejuvenate one's soul while another may view it as a miserable, gloomy, and hopeless day. Truth is just a matter of perspective.

It takes a lot of effort to step out of your perceptive truth to view someone else's truth, but it is possible and worth the work. For when you do, relationships with others as well as with yourself become less of a struggle, and they even can be fun.

If you fight against the experience of new perspectives, then feelings of vulnerability and fear arise. This is often because some sort of change is involved, and change can produce resistance to the unknown.

Fear: Anticipation of Misfortune or Pain

Even today the horrific tragedy of September eleventh has affected millions of people, not only by taking the lives of loved ones, but it continues to shake our "safe boxes" that we so strategically manipulate to fit our personal needs and wants. Suddenly the life we had accepted as truth was viciously torn apart, leaving the feelings of vulnerability, fear, and lack of control.

Dave, 39: Tension in the Air

I hurried into the airport, expecting to be met with the usual lengthy lines of impatient people and agitated security clerks. As soon as I walked through the sliding doors, I knew something was not right. There were so few people in line and only one check-in clerk stood rigid and stiff behind the counter. Tension was in the air and it crept up the back of my neck, causing the hair on my arm to stand erect. The local TV crew passionately conversed in front of many large cameras. I glanced around nervously and wondered if maybe I missed some event. Then it hit me. It was September 11th. My ticket was booked for September 11th, 2007. The amount of apprehension I felt lingering in the airport that day was extremely uncomfortable. I even felt a bit edgy, but the flight that day proved uneventful.

It is during these times—when we feel most vulnerable—that can be the best time to grab fear by the horns and embrace it. Contradictory to how it feels when you're in the midst of a struggle, fear and vulnerability are not bad things. These natural feelings are actually gifts in disguise. Fear wakes you up, challenges what you believe, and pushes you to see—beyond your comfort zone—into a world of infinite possibilities.

A keyword associated with fear is anticipation. Walking down a dark alleyway is not as frightening as walking the alley and knowing that someone is there watching you, ready to jump out at any given second. The anticipation of knowing this can be nerve-racking.

Just like in the movies, right before the shark attacks the swimmer with its menacing jaw, suspenseful music shakes the theater and the anticipation of what is to come grows within you, building your emotions to a climax.

Man's fear is surpassing man's experience of his passion for living; fear has become his dominant motivator, and his biggest obstacle.
—Chea Hetaka

Contemporary society has left behind much of its innate sanity and replaced it with fear. We see this in newspapers, our bureaucracies, our offices, high in the skies, in parents warnings to their children, and everywhere else around us. It has become common and ingrained as a truth—via the media, the mood of the world, and our own mistakes and disappointments. Fear can keep us from taking risks, from pursuing those challenges that promote growth and learning, and from experiencing a lot of fun.

When I was six years old, I experienced my first downhill skiing adventure and I don't remember it being a particularly pleasant experience. My nose was red and frosty, my skis slipped in every direction except for parallel to each other, and my bottom was black and blue for days. The second time I made an attempt at skiing was with an enthusiastic boyfriend whose regular mode of exercise was extreme. Leaving the safety of the chair lift, I fell backward and my head met the wooden chair with a sharp thud, which forcefully threw me forward onto my knees where my bottom then met the wooden bench with a solid smack. I was left sprawled out, face first, on the icy snow. After ten minutes of struggling just to stand on those slippery, obnoxious skis, I succeeded. At the top of the mountain I finally stood, gripping my poles with white knuckles, and yes, it was only the miniscule bunny slope, but to me it was as if we were high on top of Mt. Lassen. Before I could appreciate my success in standing, I found myself sliding, slipping and racing down hill at tremendous speed. Not even my radical boyfriend could keep up with me this time.

This could have been a joyous moment while racing at top speed with the wind licking my chilled face, but I only felt my heart ferociously palpitating and my legs shaking violently. My eyes stared at the lodge, which was coming closer and closer. Many people hastily dodged out of the way when they saw a frantic woman flailing her arms wildly. With a look of terror frozen on my face, I speed down the hill at Olympian speed.

Needless to say, I made a record time, landing inches before the lodge with a somersaulting crash, skis flying every which way. I physically escaped with only a twisted right ankle.

The loss of control felt during my ski extravaganza stayed with me for twelve years and I was terrified of downhill skiing. Never did I try it again until the day our family decided on a ski trip. I had planned to read in the comfort of the warm lodge. In the car, on the way to the mountains, my seven-year-old daughter questioned, "Mama, if you give up trying, how will you ever be able to ski with me?" Children often see things with a simple eye that challenge the set mature-like adult ways with an uncertainty that is quite humbling. She had a valid point. How could I rightfully argue? I watched the snowflakes hit the windshield with blinding fury and I wondered: If I give up at this, what else am I avoiding and what other fun adventures am I missing out on? More importantly, how can I rightfully tell my children to strive for what they want to accomplish and encourage them to never give up when, I, myself, am a devotee of fear?

There are multiple reasons for my fear of skiing. In this case, the fear came from the lack of control I had felt, the fear of getting hurt, the disbelief in myself that I could learn it, and the fear of looking like a flailing fool. In reality, it was not so much the memory of the physical pain that prevented me from enjoying this sport; it was the mental contortion of this event that, over many years had magnified, twisted and manifested into my mind as a true fear.

To the mind that is still, the whole universe surrenders.
—Lao Tzo

That day I tried skiing again. It took two-and-a-half hours to ski one run down the bunny slope; but I did it and then I did it again and again. When facing a fear, there is a sense of freedom created that is naturally empowering and inspiring. When someone feels fear, it is very real to that person. She or he breathes fear, lives fear, and ultimately becomes fear, if it is not addressed. But fear is not that powerful. It is a lot like a gun; without ammunition a gun can do no harm; but once it is loaded, it can be lethal. For fear to be powerful it must be loaded, feeding off the mind's insecurities and inability to believe or have faith. It is those who do not admit feeling fear who generally fear the fear itself. Active fear makes your legs wobble, decreases your reaction time, affects eyesight and limits fine motor skills. It can consume the whole of your mind and body, or it can challenge you to succeed.

Fear is only as powerful as you let it become.

Be aware of the fears in your life. First, identify your fears and beliefs by writing them down on a notepad or journal when they surface. What do you wish to change? What is holding you back from following through with a dream or passion? What makes you sad, angry, or react? When your fears come up, read your answers to these questions and try to understand the fear, but do not over-analyze it. If we can identify our failure factor, the reoccurring fear that resurfaces as some form of blockage, we can then work with the fears by understanding it and ultimately letting it go.

You can be your own best friend or your worst enemy. There is darkness that lingers inside each of us, nudging, or perhaps jabbing, at the luminosity that radiates throughout mankind. It can be labeled evil and good, light and dark, or right and wrong, but whichever label you use is not important. Simply keep in mind that there is a flip side to everything and everyone. Even though we all possess gifts and beauty, no one is immune to violence or crime, and we all can be made culprits by our own fear, anger, addictions, and judgments.

It is refreshing to note that along with our failure factors, each one of us also possesses a success factor. Similar to the failure factor, we must first identify our own success factors before we can attempt to have an understanding of what helps us move forward. What is your own natural ability? What are your gifts? What makes you happy? What is your passion? Again, writing your answers and thoughts down on paper may seem too simple, but this can be a useful tool for years to come. Once you know your success factor, help others identify theirs and continue to pass it on. Remember, it is all based on the individual's judgment and perceptions. This step-by-step approach can lead to understanding better how you think and act, and who you become.

Judgment: The Act of Criticizing

Defined by Webster's Dictionary, "judgment" means to make a critical determination, to estimate the value or magnitude of anything.

Judgments are a normal thought process in human behavior. Try for one day to eliminate judgment. It is interesting to simply take a walk and count how many times a judgment pops up. It might surprise you to learn the volume and sometimes the intensity of thoughts and judgments that pass through the mind—about other people, things surrounding you, or about yourself. Judgments are not going to ever go away, but we can learn to let them flow through us rather than become stuck within the mind's chatter.

I can be more stubborn than the crankiest old mule, especially after attending a seminar that focused primarily on judgment. My dear friend, teacher, and extreme button-pusher, Ondre, instructed such a class. Afterwards, when I got home, I collapsed on my bed with a full-blown migraine that rushed me into the bathroom, continuously, to regurgitate. The severe flu-like symptoms were a complete contrast to the healthy and vibrant body I had been accompanied by earlier that morning before class started. My awful symptoms lasted four hours. However, my mind, still boggled by self-judgments and expectations that were brought to my attention during the class, continued to pound in my head like an active volcano. This was a concrete, heads-on experience of how we can create our own drama, illusions, headaches, victimizations, illnesses, and manipulations. I was shown both the mind's unquestionable magnitude as well as its powerfully destructive potential.

*In every encounter or experience, there is the potential for gaining
enlightenment, the possibility of finding that one missing piece
of the puzzle that brings about illumination. It is our own mind
that determines the experience.*

—Masaaki Hatsumi, 34th Ninja grandmaster

Anger: A Strong Feeling of Grievance and Displeasure

In the eighteenth century, a British physician, John Hunter,
had an exceptionally bad temper and, not surprisingly,
suffered from a heart disorder called angina pectoris. He
was known for often saying, "My life is at the mercy of
any scoundrel who chooses to put me in a passion." This
proved quite prophetic as he went to a board meeting at
St. George's Hospital in London. He was involved in a
heated argument, walked out and dropped dead.

Anger can make you the victim. It is natural for most
children to experience a temper tantrum—until about age
three or four. That, however, does not stop many of us
from remaining prey to our active tempers all our lives.

> **When you allow someone else's behavior to
> make you angry, you become the victim.**

Your mood is being ruled by the memory of the person
or event you are angry with and not by you. You are no
longer in control of your emotions at this point.

Anger is a powerful energy; it's incredibly persuasive
and awfully contagious. It can fuse your mind and soul,
causing a block that builds with pressure until it suddenly
bursts in elongated occurrences or in an explosion that
shoots uncontrolled rage. As with any emotion, anger can

limit your outlook on life, gnaw at your bones, weaken the immune system because of the stress it causes, and limit your ability to function fully.

Journal Entry: The Power of Anger
January 2004

"I turn toward anger as a form of protection when I feel weak, hurt, or scared. I turn toward anger when I feel vulnerable and the rage creates a false sense of power and control. I sit in Ondre's Victorian house, leaning forward with arms propped on my knees, fuming with anger as his presence alone catalyzes the frustrations, propelling more fury toward the surface. I cannot recall the conversation, but suddenly I do feel scared at how much I enjoy this addictive anger.

"Although people do not describe me as an angry person, I cannot deny the draw I feel toward the wicked side of this potent emotion that can feel indomitable and almighty. I see his mouth move, forming words of some kind, but all I can think of is how good it would feel to dive head first through the window and hear the shattering of broken glass. It is this night that I realize just how destructive I have let this anger become. It feels powerfully addictive and dominating. God, please, I pray to you, please help me release this anger so I can feel you again and live with peace."

Time and time again I have witnessed people who feverishly place Ondre on a grand pedestal, with the delusional thoughts that he is beyond human emotions because of the constant support he provides for others and his extraordinary connection with Spirit. This was his reply when I asked him if he ever felt angry.

"Yes, of course, and I deal with it and let it go. What

is the point of being depressed or angry for lengths of time? What is it going to achieve? If you hang on to anger, you are just being self-centered and the anger then becomes all about you. Most people who behave angrily around you want the focus to be more about them, and they desire some kind of attention. Instead of the angry person telling you want they want, they make a whole drama first before telling you want it is they want. It is a bit like people who must have a drink before they can talk to their date."

Often the source of our anger is a combination of many different aspects or situations in life, so that it becomes difficult for an individual to understand the genuine cause of the emotion when it first surfaces. Anger is often the feeling we experience when events are not going according to our plans. We create an inner idea of how things, people and events should be; and when they don't march to our tune, we get angry and either feel frustrated or try to change them. Two common avenues of anger are exceedingly pent-up frustration and self-hatred.

Anger in our society is looked upon as scary, potentially threatening, negative, and certainly not ladylike. On the flip side, anger can be an incredible driving force that can propel you forward. Anger is a natural emotion. To be a spiritual person does not mean you have to be free of anger, but the significance lies in the ability of how we deal with it.

It is not the anger alone that destroys; it is the choice of how you handle your anger, how you project it, how you deal with it, and whether you listen to it. Anger can tell you a lot about yourself and others around you. It can be a tool—or a self-destructive weapon.

When anger is used in a positive manner during physical self-defense, it can be a guard, serving you with power, strength, and protection. Even in a person considered passive, the anger that manifests can be shaped into a means of assertive behavior. The positive power of anger can encourage an individual not to give in or give up.

When anger is strong, a person may feel "blocked" by this heavily dosed emotion, which makes assessment of the situation difficult. For example, two-year-olds who are angry (sometimes even a twenty-two or forty-two-year-old), clench their hands, scrunch their face, holler, and stamp their feet. All this emotion takes over the body and mind for that moment and they no longer are open to other avenues for resolving the issue.

> **Anger can cloud judgment and produce a slower reaction time that prevents a fast and effective escape.**

Anger may stem from childhood, past or current relationships, or perhaps as far back as past lives, but it is not of great importance where the anger started. What matters is how you handle it in this present moment. The secret to dealing with anger is to receive it without judgment, to neither resist it nor own it. Don't let it impair your attitude. Let it propel you in a focused manner and watch the power evolve. The choice is yours—whether or not to become the victim.

Emotions are a game we all play and seldom win.
—Ondre

Habit: An Action That Becomes a Pattern of Behavior

A habit is an action that is repeated so often that it becomes typical, although the person with the habit may be unaware of it.

Vanessa 42: Hitting Bottom

"I made a crucial decision that shaped many of the years to come. My activity was to party. This party behavior steadily became more addictive and more difficult to escape. Being young, I was skeptical of anything that elders told me about the use of one drug leading to another. Before I knew it, my heavy drinking lead to pot, pot lead to cocaine, and the progression extended far beyond my control.

Friends were not really friends at this point, and I was not really a friend. The so-called friends around me went from snorting to freebasing cocaine and, at twenty years old, I overdosed on cocaine.

My heart was racing abnormally and my left arm became numb, lasting for hours. I grabbed my dog and held on to him, waiting…waiting, hanging on to life and knowing that I could die at any moment. I was in serious trouble, but not even my partying friend would acknowledge my overdose; she left me on the floor, lying in a panic. There is a certain level of friendship, things to hide, or not being capable of helping others in a situation like this. I knew I had hit bottom, and I was scared.

I stopped cocaine use after this episode for about a year, but I did not quit drinking. Then I went back to my habit of mixing alcohol with cocaine. I grew desperately unhappy, but the temptation was all around me, and the cocaine was usually free. Each early morning around three or four a.m., the birds started to sing outside my window. When I had to go to work, and I had been up partying all night, the bird's song became an ugly reminder of another day. I was sick and tired of telling myself the same old lies that I'm not going to do it again, but again and again, my vicious addiction of alcohol and cocaine consumption was more powerful than me.

One night, after partying with others, I hit a turning point. This is not the norm and I consider myself very lucky. After stating out loud how sick I was of this addiction—a heartfelt expression—as if a prayer came down through my head and filled my body with a healing warmth. It was like a spiritually clean light—a ray of sunlight beaming within me. This experience changed my life. I felt cleansed. I worked with different therapists and rehab programs to ensure my stability. I am eternally grateful for the ability to make a different choice and choosing to take action.

If I were to give any advice to those in a similar situation, it would be to seek help. People don't believe they can change, and then the people around you don't believe you can change, and it becomes very destructive. New friends, therapists, and rehab programs can offer a different view. Talk to people, get in a rehab program, and attend AA meetings, because the people there can believe in you when you can't believe in yourself. Then, when you are ready to believe in yourself, you have support."

Habit is either the best of servants or the worst of masters.
—Nathaniel Emmons

Without habit formation, we would have to act spontaneously on every occasion or deliberately think out what we are about to do and decide each time how to do it. Can you imagine getting dressed and undressed every day without having learned the habit of doing so? Or performing at work, driving the car, brushing your teeth, stopping for a red light? Human life without habits would be a nightmare.

> **The irony is: we make our habits.
> Then they turn around and make us.**

Overeating, procrastinating, smoking, mismanaging money, watching too much TV, being chronically late, nail biting, using drugs, lying, stressing out—this is a small list of potentially bad habits. Are you a coffee drinker? As a society, we have become more and more dependent upon the consumption of things outside us to make us feel good. Are you a person who must drink a cup of coffee in the morning in order to function properly? A cup in moderation is no big deal, but if you let a beverage determine whether your morning is going to start out happy or grumpy, maybe your habit has turned into a more serious addiction. Are you really going to give away your ownership of attitude to a cup of java? There are those who are stimulated by the passion they have for life and those who have to be stimulated to feel stimulated or to feel any passion at all.

Bad habits chip away at the life you could be living right now. They stifle the chance for success, and hold you back from enjoying rewarding personal relationships. Habits prevent you from looking and feeling great. If you want to change a bad habit, you have to first understand that you do indeed have one, and then admit it. If you admit it, then you have already taken the first step.

> **Rather than wiping your habit out of existence and leaving a gaping empty hole, try to replace your habit with something new and positive. It's helpful to not focus on the "not doing," and to think instead about "doing."**

Instead of thinking how you are missing out on that piece of chocolate cake, think of how good you will feel about taking a walk without all that sugar. Don't beat yourself up if you slip from your plan, for that can become a nasty habit on its own. Take, for example, someone who's trying to lose weight. It's a vicious cycle for those who slip, beat themselves up for bingeing, then feel worse about themselves, so they resort to eating even more food—often because it simulates emotional support and restores a false sense of self-control.

Habits are about rhythm, following a pattern of stimulus and response. What can trigger a habit is an emotion, an event, or the passing of time. Break the rhythm and you will break the habit. One way you can change the rhythm is by doing the act at different times or for different reasons. For example, try eating a chocolate bar when you really don't want one, or try not watching television when you really want to. Once you remove the mental correlation of the act with the stimulus, the act is then done by your choice, not from habit.

Habits and addictions become intermingled in the cycles of how we live, how we perceive ourselves and everything around us. This is why there is no quick fix to simple habits or severe addictions. The cycle does not necessarily have to be completely broken, but it does need to be redirected with positive habits. Cycles are a natural occurrence, around us and within us. To mention a few cycles—the changing of seasons, birth, life, death, and the hormonal cycle. Many women look at their menstrual time of month as a severe inconvenience, and their partners may try to hide as they watch hormonal demons emerge from the most secret of corners, sometimes even surprising the woman herself. But this incredibly natural cycle is a chance for a woman to shed old blood physically if not pregnant, and it is an opportunity to clear, let go, and cleanse mentally.

For those women who may get a little edgy, obnoxiously tearful, grumpy, or horrifically angry a few days prior to your menstrual period, instead of lying on the couch, slamming doors or yelling at those around you for the most insignificant reasons, try something new. There are massive amounts of energy you feel when you are more open during this premenstrual time, as everything you have been experiencing over the past month is climaxing before releasing. It is during this time that using your creative talents can be a helpful tool in keeping more balanced, as well as producing some profound pieces of art, writing, dances, or other creative activity. Don't keep all that energy bottled up. Without judgment on your creative project, let it flow. Release and redirect the energy into something positive and productive.

Men have cycles too, periods that do not physically release the discharge of blood, of course, so they may not be as apparent as those of a female cycle. It may, at first, seem that a man's life is easier. But in a way it may be more challenging for a man because he doesn't have the physical component to place blame on, so it can be a little trickier to notice when that cycle arises.

A friend, Russell, shared with me that every month he felt a tension growing, which he thought was stress piling on top of him and weighing him down. He didn't know how to release this pressure and as it climaxed, he said that he started to pick at his wife until she became grumpy with him, and it resulted in a heated argument. After the argument, Russell felt rejuvenated. He observed that the argument helped him talk and actually released all the tension. This was great, but he eventually took up woodworking as a means of release and relaxation rather than arguing with his wife.

Everyone's cycles will be different depending on the individual, but by close observation, perhaps keeping a detailed journal, you can become more aware of your cycles, addictions, and habits. Start taking preventative action through observation.

A negative attitude can become a habit, too. If you think or say negative thoughts throughout the day, this can have a negative effect on your wellbeing. Someone who frequently says, "I'm so tired," is putting out that energy—and becomes tired. Someone who repeatedly moans, "I can't do it" or "I'm so stupid," is abusing him—or herself verbally, even if laughing while saying it. Think positively. Talk positively. Become positive. Feel a positive change!

> **It's time to break habits and cycles that continually threaten the existence of inner passions and enthusiasm for living a life of fulfillment.**

What you say and think about yourself can adversely affect how your body reacts to you. A positive mental perspective and knowledge of the body's' physical abilities begin to work together in harmony rather than contradicting each other. Much like the disparity of the mind, as discussed in the next chapter, the body also can

Chapter Nine

The Body as a Weapon

It is not how much force we apply, it is in how much we believe and how true our intentions are.
—Ondre

Without a spoken word, a painted mime, dressed in black and white overalls can make a crowd burst into fits of hysterical laugher. Through his actions, in the next moment, he can transform the crowd completely into a solemn, somber state that might be better accepted at a funeral before yet another outburst of laughter consumes the crowd.

People gauge our personalities ninety percent of the time through our body language. We are all mimes who constantly give out information daily to our friends, family, and even strangers. In an intimate relationship, body language plays an especially important role in communication. In the workplace, no matter what profession, watching body language helps decipher what kind of people we are dealing with and how best to approach them.

Each day is like going on a job interview. Even if you dress the part with slacks and a tie, or a skirt and high heels, if you walk into an interview with eyes lowered, shuffled footsteps, and carrying little enthusiasm, you might as well plaster the scratched words "low self-confidence" on your forehead. Confidence does not proclaim itself as part of all of us, and it can be hard work to store it up, but a good starting point is to begin walking, talking, and moving with intent. If this sounds backwards—that you first should have the confidence and then show it—try something new today. Even if you lack confidence, go out into the world and act self-assured, and then observe people's actions towards you. Do they treat you differently or the same? Do they get angry as your strength of character develops? Or do they become more alive and motivated around you? How does it make you feel?

Do not be discouraged if people around you don't take well to your change to self-assured body language and actions. Often it provokes those closest to us because it takes them out of their comfort zone and triggers a clear perception of their own behaviors, both positive and negative. Although it may feel challenging, you can pat yourself on the back because you now know you are inspiring change—and change can lead to renewed vision and growth.

When you are about to go on a job interview, you may get pumped up, raise your confidence, show that you look and feel good through your body language and be ready to win that job. But how often do we really interview? An eerily surprising thought is that we may be interviewed far more than we think.

Assailants are keen observers. They watch your body language, how you carry and present yourself. How do you project yourself in the world? How much personal information is unknowingly shared? Opposite from an employer who chooses you for the job because of your powerful presence, an assailant picks those who are weak and vulnerable—those who they think they can easily dominate. An attacker or abuser wants an easy victim. Don't be an easy victim.

Remember, there is a flip side to everything. Just as you can be observed, you can observe as well. Often someone with ill intentions may say something or smile sweetly, but his or her body language may show adverse intentions. Maybe his body is stiff and rigid, he keeps tapping his fingers or shaking his leg up and down, or his eyes are darting around uncomfortably. If you have children, you know exactly what I mean. Ask a child who took the cookie from the cookie jar and they all shout, "Not me!" But someone with wide eyes will be fidgeting nervously! Or, as we discussed with domestic violence, an abuser often says one thing but does another. Signs like these should raise a warning flag.

We all have different life situations to deal with, and it would be nearly impossible to be on "super interview behavior" constantly. Home is where you can relax, slouch on the couch, cry while eating a pint of Ben and Jerry's ice cream, pick your nose, download the day or zone out in front of the TV. But when you walk out into that world, keep your eyes up, walk with confidence, and show through your body language that you are not to be messed with. Something as simple as this could save your life.

Physical Self-Defense:

- Stance
- Voice
- Kicks
- Hand Strikes

Described below are three kicks and three hand strikes that are easy to use by almost every person of any age, body build, or ability. The body can show weakness and it can be the choice weapon for defense. We will also discuss common ways to be grabbed and choked. The information shared in this book is meant as a guide and though it should be taken seriously, it should not take the place of a hands-on self-defense course.

Stances

Stances in the martial arts are usually set low to serve as a solid, balanced foundation for the strikes or kicks to be executed from. In training, this can be a test of strength and endurance. In preparing for self-defense, the stance need not be low to the ground, but simply one foot should be placed slightly behind the other to aid in balance. This stance gives the attacker less of a target area to work with if fists, knives, or guns are involved. From a standard standing position, even with two feet solidly on the ground, a person is easily pushed backwards and off balance. With one foot back, the shoulder turns slightly, and no longer is the body face-on to the attacker. This adds protection for the vital organs and increases quick mobility for shuffling the feet rather than cross stepping and potentially tripping over your own feet.

There is a bonus to this stance that comes in handy if someone is not physically threatening, but intruding on your space, talking at ferocious speed and trying to dump an entire day of drama on you. Simply place one foot behind you or, if needed, take one step back. Watch the difference in how you feel as this rush of drama passes right by instead of hitting you head-on like a freight train from hell.

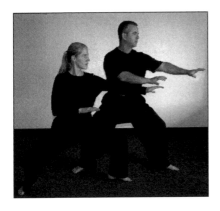

Martial Arts Stance

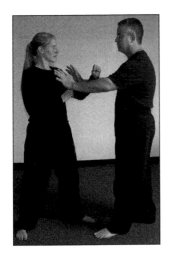

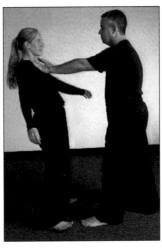

One Foot Back Stance

Face-On Stance

The Power of Voice

Statistics show that we get ninety percent of what we ask for, if only we have the guts to utilize our voice—and ask. Using the voice is natural for some and grueling for others. You might perceive it as difficult if you were raised in the era when children should be seen but not heard, or if you were ridiculed when you spoke, or became afraid to say "no" because a guilty conscience evolved into ruthless self-blame. Whatever the reason, do not be afraid to use your voice, but remember to keep your words positive.

The importance of voice is critical in defensive circumstances. First, it is intimidating and surprising to the opponent if you start yelling boisterously. Second, when your voice is added to a defensive movement, it helps support the intent to focus and follow through when utilizing a physical technique. Third, if you get hit in the stomach area and the wind gets knocked out, if you yell, exhale or "kiap up," you can maintain your air supply and continue defending yourself.

With all hand strikes and kicks, remember to combine your technique with an added "kiap," or simply yell "No!" The power of the voice is one of our best defenses and helps to strengthen the mind/body correlation.

Kicks: Encouraging Balance

There are numerous kicks—front leg kicks, back leg kicks, spin kicks, jumping kicks, and flying kicks. But rest assured we will leave those fancy, flying, over-the-top of houses tricks to Hollywood. The high kicks are an art of the body, beautiful, strong, and they demonstrate flexibility, but for self-defense, the kicks are kept below the waist, encouraging balance and leaving the torso for hand strikes. The front snap kick, stomp kick, and knee kick may not be the most impressive looking, but they are simple, fast, and effective. With any of these kicks, the front or back leg can be used. In general, the front leg has more speed and the back leg has more power.

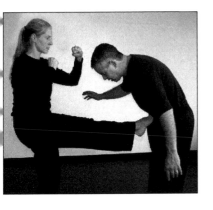

Front Snap Kick

Front snap kick can be executed with or without shoes on. With shoes on, kick the leg as if shooting a goal in the world Olympic soccer game—hard and fast. Without shoes, the toes curl upward and, with a locked ankle, the point of contact is the ball of the foot. The foot snaps out—hard, fast, and powerful.

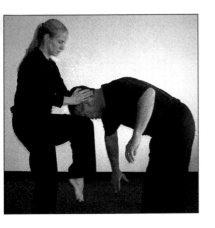

Knee Kick

Grab the head and, pulling with a downward motion, bring the knee up with a powerful thrust into the opponent's face. Or grab the shoulders and bring the knee to the stomach or groin.

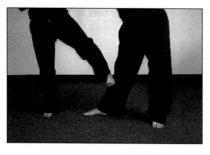

Stomp Kick

Just as the term "stomp kick" sounds, simply lift your foot and stomp down as hard as you can, using the entire bottom surface of your foot. You can put your weight into this kick for added pressure.

Hand Strikes: Effective and Powerful

Fast action from the hip will give any hand strike a potency advantage; however, these strikes can be rendered from any angle. Although simple in form, do not underestimate the forceful puissance of these strikes. Keep in mind that it may take three, four, five, maybe ten strikes before escaping. Do whatever it takes to get free.

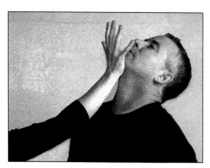

Palm Strike

Face your hands together and tap the hard part of your palms together. This should give you some idea of how effective this strike can be. Open fingers wide allowing internal energy to pass through, then, making a strong wrist, strike with your palm against your target. With most hand strikes, it is best to keep a slight bend in the arm to keep from hyper-extending the elbow. If you are practicing these strikes for the first time, do them slowly with less power before executing a full-force blow, to ensure proper technique.

Hammer Fist

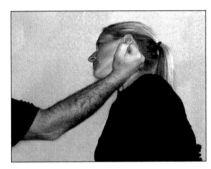

With a tight fist, make sure your thumb is securely set against the outside of your fingers. If the thumb stays upright or is placed inside your fist it could easily be broken. The striking area is on the pinky side of the hand (or knife-edge), although both sides can be used. The bigger the circle made with your arm, the more power the strike delivers. Use the same motion as if hammering and driving a nail through a two-by-four.

Hammer fist is also known as the "anger management" strike. Why? Try it and find out. All you need is a pillow, bed, or couch. Use hammer fist technique with any pent-up frustrations or anger, and save money on a therapist.

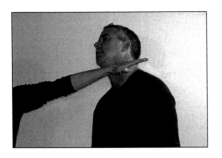

Chop

Bringing your hand to your opposite shoulder, make a strong forearm with an open hand and tightly closed fingers. Again, the thumb is tucked close to the fingers to aid in support and to avoid breakage. Palm should face downward. This is a powerful strike that can also be performed in an up-and-down motion as if chopping a piece of wood.

Escape Techniques

There are as many ways of being grabbed or accosted, as there are ways of escaping. Discussed below are some possible grabs focused on using escape techniques that do not require the use of victim muscle power. The focus is placed on the attacker's vulnerability's and how the victim might use the attacker's weaknesses to their advantage. Remember, if you are being attacked, it is because you appear weak to the assailant. Prove the attacker wrong, immediately. You have the element of surprise on your side for a limited amount of time. Don't lose it—use it—and act quickly. If the assailant is trying to move you to a car, do whatever you can to avoid being moved. An old school of thought is to play along as though weak until there is a chance for escape. Today, we know that if an assailant wants you inside a vehicle, he/she has plans to move you to an isolated spot where there will be less of a chance of being caught. That means less of a chance for you to get help. Act now, and be safe now.

You can run if there is somewhere safe to run to, like a restaurant, grocery store, or neighbor's home. If there is nothing around, the assailant must be disabled enough to give you time to run for help.

Remember, there are endless possibilities for how one can be grabbed or accosted, but we will cover a few of the most common grabs and the best means of escape. Again, this should not stop you from attending self-defense classes. This material is intended as an introduction guide and is coefficient with most beginner-level Safety Awareness Training classes offered.

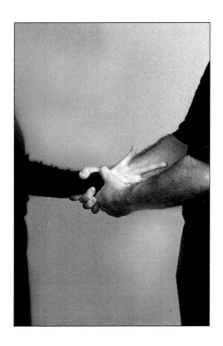

**Wrist Escape #1-Assailant grabs
one wrist with two hands**

The most common response if grabbed aggressively is to pull away in a backward motion. This makes the assailant pull harder the opposite way, creating an even tighter grip. Instead of pulling away, step forward toward the assailant, catching him by surprise and throwing him off balance. Bring your hand up through the thumb and forefinger. Think of pushing your elbow up toward his face to ensure an effective follow through that does not require muscle strength alone.

A crucial point: Do not try to pit your strength against that of the attacker. Instead focus on using the weaker part of his anatomy, which is the grip of the thumb and forefinger. Though it is hard to escape from a tight grip of four fingers, the weakest link is where the thumb meets the fingers.

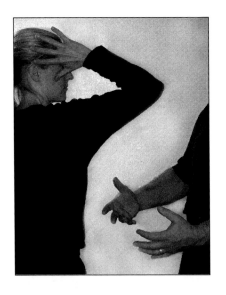

**Wrist Escape #2–Assailant grabs
mirroring hand wrist with one hand**

Step forward, this time bring your hand, with palm facing down, to your opposite shoulder. The fingers should be wide open, allowing energy to pass and the forearm remains strong.

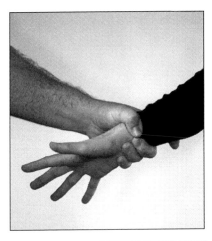

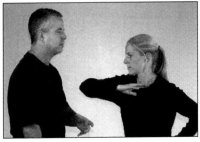

Wrist Escape #3–Assailant grabs opposite wrist with one hand

Step forward and extend hand with an upward motion, while rotating palm face up and over the assailant's opposite shoulder, releasing the opponent's grip.

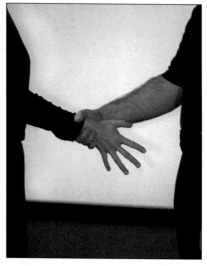

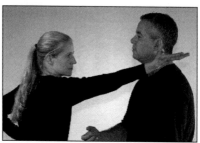

**Choke Hold – The assailant is facing
the victim and grabs with two hands while tightly
squeezing around the victim's neck.**

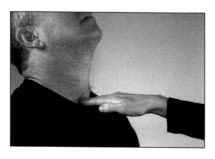

With any chokehold, the first and foremost concern is the limited conscious time that remains before passing out. There are many chokeholds and choke escape techniques that require considerable practice and detailed technique, both of which should be learned in a hands-on self-defense class.

But this technique is simple, extremely effective, and should not be tried in play. Push your thumb or fingers into the attacker's throat below the Adam's apple where there is an indentation. This requires little strength on your part. With force push straight back. With this technique, your attacker can experience temporary air loss, drowning from internal bleeding, or a collapsed esophagus.

In chapter ten, we will cover the main target areas of the body. These are the vulnerable places of the body where kicks and hand strikes will prove most effective.

Chapter Ten

Target Areas

The ultimate measure of man is not where he stands in moments of comfort and convenience, but where he stands at times of challenge and controversy.
—Martin Luther King, Jr.

During my first martial arts demonstration I stood in front of a large crowd of children, adults, and families. I practiced the ladies' self-defense demo many times, but with this many eager eyes, I secretly wished I could hide in the ladies' bathroom. Before I could plan my escape route, my demo partner came running fiercely toward me, all two hundred and twenty pounds, ready to attack and hollering profusely. Suddenly my legs buckled, and my eyes widened like a blinded deer stupefied by headlights. As planned he picked me up, leaving my legs dangling. Instantly I opened both of my hands and met his ears with a mighty crack. As he dropped to the floor, I knew I had hit directly over his ears, instead of above them as we are supposed to do for demo purposes to avoid the real effect of a busted eardrum.

Wow, it really does work, I thought to myself! Luckily I pulled back quickly and did not follow through with the movement. From his extensive martial arts background, my partner resumed position quickly and once again came yelling and running toward me with what I thought was, just maybe, a little more aggression the second time around.

The martial arts can include joint locks, pressure points, and various detailed techniques, as well as weapons that work incredibly well in self-defense or in disabling an assailant. However, not everyone has the time or desire needed to master this form of discipline.

It is highly recommended that you practice the techniques as often as possible to help with muscle memory. If time is spent on these techniques, strikes, and kicks, then— if attacked—your response will be instinctive as your body's muscle memory enables an immediate reaction.

Due to busy schedules and a variety of priorities, the list of target areas below is simplified so it can be read and used today, and remembered for tomorrow. A person of almost any age or ability can use these techniques if you focus, not on hitting a precise pressure point or learning a direct angle of joint lock, but simply striking to the most vulnerable areas of the body.

The Body's Most Vulnerable Target Areas

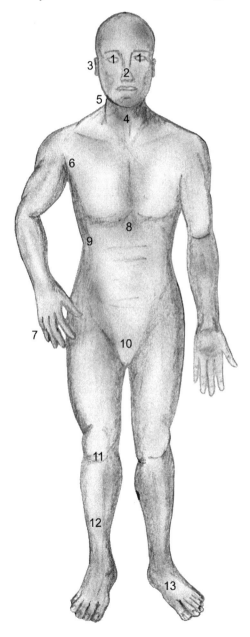

1. The eyes are without a doubt extremely sensitive to even the slightest touch. Eyes are easy to poke with fingers, keys, or other sharp objects. It is possible to push in and pop an eyeball out with the thumb or fingers. The elasticity of the intrinsic muscles makes it easy to poke the eyeball out of the orbital fissure with little effort on your part.

2. Palm strike or hammer fist into the nose can cause confusion, pain, tearing of the eyes, or nasal bleeding. If shoved at a forty-five degree angle, it could easily result in death by forcing the septal cartilage through the internal portions of the nose and through the crista galli into the assailant's brain.

3. Palm strike repeatedly over the ears with one hand or both hands, pull ears straight down and off, or stick pencil, stick, or something sharp into the ear. The ears can yield a variety of immobilizing effects as the air is easily trapped in the external acoustic meatus and forced down into the eardrum. The eardrum can rupture, causing much pain, loss of hearing, and bleeding from the mouth, ear, and into the throat through the internal auditory tube. A sufficient or continued blow to the ears can also cause loss of equilibrium.

4. A chop or any direct strike is effective on the throat. Because of the vital functions of the esophagus, larynx, and thyroid cartilage, the internal portions of the anterior neck region are crucial targets. Any swelling in the area will cut the air supply to the windpipe and blood drowning is also likely where sufficient force is applied.

5. Chop to either side of the neck (called the sterno-cleidomastoid region). There is much more here than meets the eye. Contraction and dizziness would be the initial response to a hit of medium

force. A blow of significant force could swell, collapse, or burst one or both of the major bloodlines whose most important function is supplying the blood transactions to the brain.

6. Although this would not be a disabling technique, for informational purposes, the inner arms and the inner thighs are much more sensitive and react to pain than the outer portions.

7. Pull back any or all fingers to release a grip or to break fingers. This is easy and effective!

8. The sternum is a flat narrow bone about six inches long situated in the centerline between the pectoralis muscles in the front of the thorax. In CPR the sternum responds well to the cardiorespiratory thrust, because the heart lies close behind the sternum. If struck as a target, the sternum can easily be broken and result in cardiorespiratory response from coughing, pain, or temporary paralysis of vital organs.

9. The pectoralis major and minor muscles protect all but the sixth through tenth ribs. So the last five ribs are our focus. Striking these ribs can produce a winding effect or, with more force, they can be broken. Note: the floating ribs cannot be struck from the front.

10. Both males and females can be attacked in the sensitive groin area using any hand strike or kick. A groin kick most often causes temporary discomfort due to the transmission of pain to the abdominal area. The pain can often turn to nausea or cramping of the abdominals. Groin strikes in some cases are effective psychologically as well as physically. Although some people have more fear in a strike to the groin, it is not as fatal as a strike to the nose.

11. The knee is one of the most vulnerable areas on the lower body. Even though it can be a weapon as well, it is a good target because of its four-way vulnerability. Stomp kick or front snap-kick into the front of the knee, the outside or inside of the knee, and to the back of the knee. If you are on the ground, you can palm strike to the knees. Even a well-built, muscular person can take only limited pressure against the knee.

12. Stomp kick the shin and slide down to the top of foot. The shin is sensitive because the bone is relatively exposed with only a little skin covering it. It is an easy target to strike, especially if you are wearing high-heeled or hard-tipped shoes.

13. Stomp kick on the top of the foot. The tarsus is the collection of bones between the tibia and metatarsus and although it is one of the body's most powerful anatomical weapons, it also serves well as a vulnerable target area. An impact to the top of the foot could prove disabling, much like the knee. The tarsus is a supportive structure and if it receives a blow, it may not be able to hold the body's weight.

Does it sound gruesome yet? Just remember, what an attacker can do to you may be much, much worse. A lady who participated in Safety Awareness Training told me with pure conviction that she by no means could or would ever be able to hit someone and poke them in the eyes. Agreeing that it sounded gruesome, but as an advocate of self-protection and a mother myself, I asked her, "Do you have any children?"

She answered proudly, "Why, yes, I have two young children."

"What would you do if you walked out of the grocery

store and someone grabbed your children and dragged them to a car?"

She suddenly jumped out of her chair, her face contorted with narrowed eyes, and the soft-spoken lady was now wildly swinging her arms around, passionately growling, "I would tear their eyeballs out, smack their ears, palm strike their nose, and take them to the ground." She gave a final huff then plopped herself down in the chair and everyone stared at her in bewilderment before an enthusiastic applaud filled the room.

If this lady will protect her children, why does she not take the same initiative and value in protecting herself? Would you? Do you believe you are worth defending?

The Danger of Knives

Within its range, a knife never runs out of ammunition, never jams, never misfires, rarely misses its target; cuts bone, tendon, muscle, arteries, and veins with one thrust. With superior concealment capabilities, it has psychological advantage as well. Within their respective ranges, knives are actually more lethal than firearms.

The terrorist attacks on the United States World Trade Center and Pentagon are a good reminder that there are times when regular people face inescapable, violent confrontations. The weapons of choice at that time were box cutters and knives with blades that were less than four inches long. According to reports, they were simple tools that could be purchased from a local hardware store.

One threat of knives, razors, or other edged weapons is the level of intimidation they create. When discussing weapons in my self-defense classes, I discovered that about half the students don't understand or consider the extreme dangers of knives, and half believe they are already doomed if ever attacked with a knife. The real threat posed by any edged weapon is penetration of the blade. If the blade pierces more than two inches into your body, it can produce lethal results. Vital organs, veins, and major arteries are in danger once there is penetration.

There are two types of knife fighters. One clearly knows what he is doing and uses his weapon as a tool to accomplish his deed. The second is a person who uses this weapon as a form of intimidation and likely would feel powerless without it.

If you do happen to get cut in an attack, do not panic. Consciously slow your breathing down, apply pressure to wounds, and elevate any limb that has been injured. If you have a chest wound, seal it and protect your airway. In case you become unconscious, you don't want to drown in your own blood. If you have a punctured lung, exhale first and use something airtight to cover and seal the wound.

When looking for an offensive/defensive knife course, make certain that the program includes awareness strategies and realistic hands-on counter tactics. I was amazed the first time I took a knife-fighting course and sliced a huge chunk of hanging cow flesh I'd purchased from the butcher next door (which alone was a challenge to my vegetarian mind). I sliced with little strength using a small 1-1/2-inch knife that hangs from my key chain. The flesh immediately separated, folding down, limp and bloody.

Attackers often use a weapon as a form of intimidation and sometimes want to attack something, however big or small, in order to feel that they did not fail. In one situation, a man who had pulled into a rest stop while traveling was violently greeted by a man with a knife. As soon as the traveler entered the restroom, the assailant thrust the knife into his side, pushed him against the sinks and demanded his wallet. The wallet was left in the car and although the man insisted he did not have it, the aggressor elevated the knife and firmly applied pressure, adamantly demanding the victim's wallet. The innocent man reached into his pocket and pulled out a dollar bill that he had stuffed in there earlier that morning after stopping at a gas mart. He held out the dollar and immediately the man extracted the knife, grabbed the dollar and ran out the door toward the woods. This traveler was lucky indeed, as knife threats are nothing to take lightly.

An attacker can sense a person's weakness and go after it effectively. A common way for anyone to get close to you is by asking a question. It seems a simple approach, but its effectiveness cannot be doubted. From early childhood, we are expected to answer promptly if asked a question. If someone near you asks you for the time, most likely you glance at your watch and give the time without giving it a second thought. First of all, be aware that you have just engaged in conversation with a potential attacker. Second, your eyes go down to your watch and for an instant you are not aware of what is happening around you. An instant is all an attacker needs to grab your wallet and run, or hurl a punch and drag you down the back alley or into a waiting car.

I am not suggesting that each time someone asks you the time of day, you break into your grounded martial arts stance ready to fight. But I do suggest that you be aware of the possible ways attackers can get close without seeming intrusive. A simple solution to the "time" question is to step back slightly, posing you in a balanced stance with less of a target area and to raise your arm to eye level so your vision is on the person, your surroundings, and the watch at the same time. This stance is also helpful if attacks involve weapons, such as a knife or gun, as it decreases the mass target area, resulting in less chance of being struck.

Another attacker approach is that of the "knight in shining armor" or the aggressor playing the role of victim and preying on the goodness in your heart. Serial killer Ted Bundy wore a cast on one arm and carried a load of law books in another. As he walked toward the law school that he was attending, he followed a fellow student, a beautiful young lady. Suddenly and on purpose, he tripped, spewing books in all directions. The young lady helped pick up his books as Bundy showed signs of difficulty in managing with his broken arm. He smiled, thanking her, and asked if she would mind carrying them over to his car, which was not far. She willingly carried them and, when they reached his Volkswagen, he opened the passenger door for her to place the books on the seat. As the young lady leaned over, placing the books down, he hit her on the back of the head, pushed her in the car and slammed the door shut. The manipulative assailant used lack of power to overcome this lady's genuine desire to help someone in need.

Criminals not only work alone but also in pairs. Bruce was at the local paint store when a beautiful young woman, who looked like she stepped out of a modeling photo shoot, walked up close to him in the aisle and kept glancing his way while fluttering her long eyelashes. Not only was Bruce distracted as he grabbed the forest green glossy paint, even though he had come for plain primer, but he had no idea that there was a man on the other side of him. That man whisked his wallet from his rear jeans pocket and the two thieves were out of the store in a flash.

Some of us let down our guard if approached by a female or a child. A crying child may approach you saying he/she is lost and ask for help. It can be in that instant where you reach down to hold the child's small hand, or kneel to comfort the child, that you receive a mighty blow to the head and wake up to find yourself victimized in an unknown location. Or a child may tell you where he/she is to meet his/her parents, and when you get to that destination you are greeted, not by thankful parents but instead by the perpetrator of a premeditated violent act for which you are suddenly a victim.

Stalkers or other criminal assailants may have a false sense of freedom and believe that they may do as they damn well please. They may see themselves as God or working through God. An assailant will try to intimidate you and use your own fears as a weapon against you.

They will use many different avenues to approach you, but what they all have in common is a desire to somehow get close to you.

After shopping in a mall, Laura gathered her newly bought items, walked out to the parking lot and found that her car had a flat tire. She placed her shopping bags in the trunk and proceeded to take out her jack and spare tire. A man approached who carried a briefcase and wore a business suit. He smiled compassionately and asked if she would like assistance, and she gratefully accepted his gracious offer. After changing the tire, replacing the jack in the trunk of the car and closing it, he asked Laura for a lift to his car now "realizing" he would be late to work.

Laura felt uneasy, but also felt compelled to help this stranger who had so willingly helped her. Luckily Laura trusted her instinct and told the man that she would gladly give him a ride, but she first had to run back into the mall because she had forgotten one very important item. After reassuring him that she would be back quickly, she ran into the mall and told security what had happened. Laura returned to her car with the security worker and found that the man had vanished. After speaking with the police, Laura learned that the air in her tire had been purposely let out. In the trunk of her vehicle was the man's briefcase, which contained duct tape, knives, and rope—all the contents for what's best known as a rape kit.

The unaware, the weak, the ill, and the faint-hearted will fall. The strong survive. The same applies to the mind and spirit. A weak mind or a fractured spirit is a beacon to those who hunt to hurt. We are all worth defending. This belief begins by finding value in your self. A person called stupid is not stupid. They only become stupid if they believe it. The more you value yourself, the less likely you are a victim.

I ask again, are you worth defending?

Chapter Eleven

Safety and Sanity

Change your thoughts and you change your world.
—Norman Vincent Peale

Stress: Mental, Emotional or Physical Strain

There are many things in life that we simply can't control, but there are few that we can't learn to manage. What do you associate with the word stress? Do your armpits get sticky? Does your stomach churn? Are you already pulling at your hair? There are as many ways to experience stress, as there are people who experience change in their lives. Stress is the way we react physically and emotionally to change and, like change, stress can be either positive or negative.

Positive stress can help you concentrate, focus and get the job done. Many people work most efficiently under this kind of stress, and the experience of this type of stress can stay positive as long as there is time to relax and enjoy the accomplishment after the challenge is met. This allows our physical and emotional reserves to rebuild and re-fortify for the next challenge headed our way.

Stress can become a constant, ongoing cycle that can harm your health and wellbeing. Many situations can "push our buttons," and for some stress is a way of life. Stress is negative when you stay "geared up" and cannot or do not know how to relax after a challenge has been met. The good news is that you can learn to manage stress so that you are in control.

Becoming aware of stress is a two-fold process. First, try to identify some small things that make you feel stressed. Perhaps you missed a bus, misplaced your car keys, or engaged in a petty disagreement. A major lifestyle change causing stress would be, for example, getting married, losing a loved one, or the birth of a new baby. A positive major lifestyle change can be a stressor because it requires you to adapt to a new or unknown situation. Once you identify your stressors, pay attention to how your body feels under stress. Do you have pounding headaches, sweaty palms, and tight shoulders? Do you become grumpy, or does your heart beat faster? In identifying how you feel, you can observe your own individual stress reaction and this awareness, in turn, is the first step in finding solutions to the problems that caused the stress in the first place.

Avoiding hassles can help eliminate some of the minor irritations that lead to chronic, negative stress. If rushing to work makes you anxious, try getting up half an hour earlier. If you feel awful about eating fast food during your busy week, prepare some healthy meals on the weekend that can be put in the freezer. Controlling stress during lifestyle change is not as hard as it sounds. When one aspect of your life changes, either positively or negatively, try to limit other changes for a while. For example, if you are newly married or a new parent, continue to do things that bring you pleasure to help keep a balance. You don't have to change your entire lifestyle because of one variable.

When stressors combine to reach the "I can't cope" level, sometimes it is best to get a little distance from your problems to figure out the most effective way to deal with them. Some decisions may require immediate attention and some may be able to wait until later, after you have cooled down and can think with a clear, quiet mind. When there is a stress overload, it helps to break the situation or project down and take one step at a time.

Once you have become aware of stress, it's time to relax! There are many techniques for relaxing, and you know you have found the right one when it works for you. One of the body's automatic reactions to stress is rapid, shallow breathing. Breathing in slowly and deeply is one way you can encourage relaxation. Since your stress response is a physical and emotional interaction, giving yourself a mental break can help your body relax as well. Try clearing your mind of all chatter, read a good book, have a massage, take a walk, or simply take a moment to stretch. A natural physical response to stress is muscle tension, and an easy way to loosen up tight muscles and combat stress is to take a yoga class, or do stretching exercises wherever you are.

> **Stress is a part of life,**
> **but it does not have to be a way of life.**

By becoming aware of what causes stress and how you feel under stress, you can be in control. Developing a positive attitude and lifestyle is a key factor in dealing effectively with stress. Positive thinking is giving yourself the go-ahead to succeed by developing an attitude of commitment, challenge, and control toward the inevitable changes of life. Adopting a positive lifestyle by participating in physical activity, eating healthy food, getting enough rest and relaxation, and following your creative passions will help you feel better about yourself and reduce your chances of developing a stress-related illness.

"Most folks are as happy as they make up their mind to be."
—Abraham Lincoln

Exercise Tips

According to the National Center for Chronic Prevention and Health Promotion, more than sixty percent of U.S. adults do not engage in the recommended amount of physical activity, and approximately twenty-five percent of U.S. adults are not active at all. (CDC Division of Nutrition, 2006)

Physical activity can benefit you today as well as in the future. Exercise has many transformational effects on the body, mind, and spirit. Every vital organ within the body is influenced by the activity of the six hundred or more muscles that form the major part of our anatomy. We cannot enjoy vital strength or organic vigor unless we use those muscles as they were designed. When there is proper exercise of muscular tissue, your entire system and its processes work more efficiently. Circulation is markedly swayed by exercise, resulting in swift blood flow from inner structures, through large blood vessels to the body's periphery and back again. There is no stagnation, and toxins are much less likely to develop in an active bloodstream.

Exercise also favorably influences the heart. From approximately four and a half months after conception in utero, the heart must contract rhythmically and force from its chambers a definite amount of blood until the last breath has been taken. As a result of prolonged inactivity, the heart's fibers become weak and incapable of withstanding strain or tension. Exercise can also help improve the digestive tract, reduce body fat, lower cholesterol, maintain bone density, increase metabolism, and reduce blood pressure. In short, exercise can decrease stress as well as negative feelings and emotions. It relieves physical and mental tensions as it brings oxygen and nutrients to the organs and contributes favorably to our wellbeing.

So, why are you not exercising enough right now? Do an infinite number of petty excuses rattle from your mouth? Did you say you don't have time in your busy schedule? Don't forget, there are one thousand, one hundred forty minutes in every day. And contrary to an antiquated belief that exercise has to be an elongated and grueling sweaty workout at the gym, a minimal thirty minutes a day for physical activity will promote a healthier body and attitude.

You may want to walk with a friend, join a group class or plan a group bike ride. If it's fun, you are more likely to stay motivated. Swim, mow the lawn, dance, study martial arts, or take a brisk walk. The key is to find the right exercise for you—perhaps a variety of exercises that you enjoy.

Safety Tips at Home

Your home is a place where hopefully you can wind-down and relax. You may not be able to escape the chores, the squeals of children, or the neighbor's barking dog, but some easy precautions can make your home a safe haven:

- Put a timer or light sensor in your entranceways. Contact your local councilperson, park official, or security officer to have lights put in dangerous areas in your neighborhood.
- Install a deadbolt that is at least one-inch deep, and be sure to change locks in a new residence.
- Install blinds or shades on windows.

- Demand identification from unexpected service people claiming to make repairs, and call the company before opening the door. Be aware of fraud.
- Teach children NOT to open the door, or give out any information over the phone or Internet.
- Install a peephole and always look through it before opening the door.

If you are not sure whether your house or apartment is secure, you can contact your local law enforcement officers and ask someone to come out and conduct a service check. The Neighborhood Watch Unit will also come to your neighborhood to discuss safety and how to be more responsive in an emergency.

Stretching Smarts

Stretching is important for all ages. Why? Stretching increases the length of both muscles and tendons. This leads to an increased range of movement and encourages limbs and joints to flex further before an injury occurs. Stretching is imperative for preventing physical injury, as well as helping to reduce stress and tension (as mentioned earlier), enhancing muscular coordination, and increasing energy and blood circulation. You can stretch on your own, get a massage that focuses on stretching the body, and/or join a yoga class. After feeling cramped or sitting for a while, we stretch naturally, and often unconsciously, because it feels good.

Nutrition in a Nutshell

Which of the following is your definition of nutrition?

Definition 1: Healthy eating means choosing a variety of foods from the basic food groups: meat or meat substitutes, dairy, fruits and veggies; grains, such as pasta and breads; and a limited amount of fats and sweets. Keep everything in moderation.

Definition 2: Healthy eating means eating as much pasta with butter as possible with unlimited snacks of potato chips and chocolate, a double cheese burger and fries at least five times a week, and absolutely no greens.

I guess it is all a matter of perspective, but I daresay that the first definition will produce a happier and healthier you. It's not always easy to get the nutrition you need when everyone is juggling busy schedules, and convenience foods are readily available. "In the past thirty years, the prevalence of excess weight and obesity has increased sharply for both adults and children. Since 1976–80, the prevalence of obesity among U.S. adults has approximately doubled. In 2005–06, more than thirty-four percent of adults aged twenty or older were obese. The prevalence of overweight among children aged 2–5 years increased from 5% during 1976–80 to 13.9% during 2003–04. During the same period, the prevalence increased from 6.5% to 18.8% among young people aged 6–11 years, and 4% to 17.4% among those aged 12–19 years." (CDC, 2008)

A healthy diet is one of the most important ways you can maintain an active lifestyle and protect against health problems. Healthy eating increases energy, improves the way the body functions, strengthens the immune system and thwarts weight gain. Paying attention to diet and exercise can effectively control weight, but if you find yourself constantly worrying about your weight and thinking about what you are or are not going to eat, you may have an unhealthy relationship with food. Sometimes eating disorders develop from obsessive attitudes about food or body image.

An eating disorder is a psychological condition that manifests in unhealthy eating habits. These habits fall onto a continuum, from eating a healthy, balanced diet on one end, to serious disorders on the other. Eating disorders are more common than expected and often, as they are secretive by nature, they can go undetected for a long time. Eating disorders produce serious emotional and physical effects that involve such disturbances as: not eating enough, repeatedly eating too much in a short period of time, or taking drastic measures to rid the body of calories consumed (purging by vomiting, overuse of diuretics or laxatives, excessive exercising, or fasting). Individual factors that may trigger eating disorders include self-esteem issues, social anxiety, stress, depression, ineffective coping issues, and feeling out of control.

There are numerous books and other resources with specific information about nutrition, exercise, and stretching. The point here is to take notice of the mind/body connection. What you do for your body will indicate what your body will do for you.

Safety on the Street

- Keep one hand free when carrying bags or books. Don't overload! You want to be able to defend yourself if need be.

- Dress for fight or flight. Fight or flight is our body's response to perceived dangers. It is our body's primitive, automatic, inborn response that prepares the body to either "fight" or "flee" from any threat to survival.

We do not have control over everything, but we can usually choose the clothes we wear. Be conscious of where you are going and how you dress. For, example, it is difficult to fight or flee from any threat in high-heeled shoes or a tight skirt. Be aware that ties and lanyards around the neck are a handy help to an assailant who is keen on choking his/her victims. Even certain fashion trends that may look cool can put you in harm's way, such as the saggy-pants style where the boxers show and pants hang well below the butt. I know a high school boy who was involved in a fight and ended up sprawled on the cement because he tripped over his very own sagging pants.

- Walk around—rather than through—groups. It is easy to become a pickpocket victim in a crowd. Someone can come close to you with a weapon and direct you out of the crowd without others noticing anything of the ordinary.
- Turn around and check behind you if you feel you are being followed. It is always better to be on the safe side. You don't have to break into your martial arts stance each time you turn to look, but stay alert. Take the time to stop, look, and listen with all your senses.
- Know where the local police station is located. Go there if you are being followed in your vehicle.
- Avoid elevators with lone people in them or groups of people who make you feel uncomfortable.

- Always have your house keys ready before you get to the door. Have your car keys ready before reaching your car. Keys can also be used as a weapon.
- Lock your automobile and look in, under, and around your car before entering.
- Never hitchhike or pick up hitchhikers; you never know who they are or what they want.
- Use the buddy system. A pair or group of people is less attractive to an assailant than someone alone. Remember they are looking for easy victims. Wait to see if your friends are safely in the house or in the car before driving away.

Most importantly, trust your intuition. If you have a gut feeling that a situation isn't safe, believe it and act upon it. Never feel too embarrassed to take evasive action. Those "gut feelings" are often indicators that a situation is dangerous.

Keep Clear, Keep Clean

All day long you are probably surrounded by people, either at work, on the phone, while grocery shopping, at the gym, or at home with your family. Other people's emotions, problems, concerns, worries, and stress fill the air. These are the days you may come home extra exhausted, worn to a frazzle, and feel an unexplained moodiness. You may feel "filled" up and don't want to hear one more word from anyone. This is your body talking to you. It's like an oil filter that's packed to the brim with dirt. It is past time to cleanse; don't ruin your engine.

Know what is inside of you, and let it go. Some cleansing techniques that I have found useful include cycle breathing, in through your mouth and out through your nose, or simply clearing your intention for a fresh day. But the most powerful cleanser of all comes through prayer and meditation.

There are several ways to cleanse the body, mind, and spirit. If you want to buy a book on cleansing methods and proceed directly from point to point—go for it. Perhaps you'd prefer to listen to music or simply take a few minutes out of your day to breathe and regroup. A quiet getaway at work, favored by many, is the privacy of a bathroom stall! I found the privacy of the bathroom at home helpful, too. Maybe you prefer taking a walk to clear your mind, creating art, reading a good book, spending time in nature, or building something. You will know what's right for you, because the right thing feels good. Any stress inside and around you will start to diminish, and your sanity will return. It doesn't matter what method you choose, just as long as you have a healthy way to clear, reconnect with yourself and restore balance between your mind and body.

To defend yourself in a physical assault, it is imperative for your safety to have an awareness of how your body works and reacts. If we are too tangled and distracted from the vigorous emotions that consume us, it is nearly impossible to remain alert or create the awareness needed to avoid potential hazards.

A balanced mind that is in tune with the body ensures a greater chance for survival.

Chapter Twelve

Take Charge of Your Life!

The time is always right to do what is right.
—Martin Luther King, Jr.

The Power of a Positive Attitude

Ultimately, you are the one in control of making changes in your life. Take a moment to step back and observe. Do you feel passionate about your occupation? Is your relationship healthy? Are you waking up with a smile on your face, or do you resort to covering your face with a pillow at the first sign of sunlight? If you are stuck in the same situation with the same unhealthy repetitive cycles popping up, it's time to make a change. Keep in mind; it looks easier at first to blame those around you. But it all boils down to you taking the responsibility to change your life. It is not your husband, your wife, your boss, cat, doctor, or garbage man's fault if you feel unhappy or inadequate.

> **Why spend your time trying to blame others when you can spend the time wisely, looking at what you can do to make a positive change in your life?**

Maybe it starts with simply waking up tomorrow morning and, instead of the usual groan, greet the day

133

with an enthusiastic, "Thank you for this beautiful day!" I can hear you mumbling already but, before you throw the book across the room, there's something you need to know. Change usually begins with doing something you don't really want to do. Do not underestimate the power of attitude. A positive attitude is essential for successful self-defense. Often we count our weaknesses rather than our abilities.

> *"If you are walking on thin ice, it either wakes you up or you drown."*
> —Ondre

Have compassion for yourself; every issue that comes up, get excited about it and see what you can learn.

> *A positive attitude causes a chain reaction of positive thoughts, events, and outcomes. It is a catalyst and it sparks extraordinary results.*
> —Wade Boggs

Living with a positive attitude is a method of self-defense that generates awareness. In turn, it takes awareness to keep that positive attitude. Imagine waking up with a gold medallion hanging around your neck. On one side there is a "P" for positive and the other side is "N" for negative. How many times does your medallion switch during the day? Maybe it starts with "P" bold and proud, but on your drive to work, someone cuts in front of you, giving you the finger. Boom! Your blood boils and the medallion suddenly switches to "Negative." It is natural for anyone's medallion to flip from side to side. You are not a failure if it boldly states "N." The key is how fast you are able to flip that medallion back to "Positive." Anyone who has been around negative people knows how draining and toxic negativity can make the atmosphere around you feel. Negative people feed off negativity, which breeds at a tremendous rate. They live for and create drama, and often feel unsatisfied when life is calm around them—to such a point that they look for things to be annoyed about. It becomes not only a part of them, but it is the fire that makes them feel alive. So it continues until it sometimes results in illness or disease.

With a positive attitude you are more likely to be centered and grounded, increasing your ability to be aware of what surrounds you. Also, people with positive attitudes tend to enjoy hanging out with like-minded individuals, decreasing the chance for undesired or even threatening conduct.

You have to be really selfish and self-centered to get involved in other people's drama because it then becomes all about you. I suppose it is people's needs that drive people to be involved in drama, but their drama is really none of your business. Some people need drama to make life more exciting, but why not just do your job?
—Ondre

A positive approach to life in general—both in your mental attitude and physical lifestyle—can help you approach life and stress as a challenge to be enjoyed. Positive thinking is giving yourself the green light to succeed. Think of how your life could change if you delete mischievous perfection, desire for control, and merciless fear, and instead develop an attitude of challenge, commitment, and flow toward the inevitable changes of life. Attitude is a choice.

The pessimist sees difficulty in every opportunity.
The optimist sees opportunity in every difficulty.
—Winston Churchill

After much contemplation, I could bare it no longer. I asked Ondre the extensively pondered over question, "What is the meaning of life?" He tilted his head slightly and looked at me seriously and then with a warm smile he said, "It is quite simple, really." I leaned closer, my eyes widening with intense anticipation. Secretly I hoped that in a couple minutes, when I embraced the true meaning of life, my past and present challenges would magically be eliminated. I stretched my neck even further as if this might help me better understand the complexity of words that I was sure this answer would hold. "Happiness," Ondre said quietly and, with a wink of the eye, he walked to the kitchen to warm the teakettle. He left me there, challenging my own mind's absorption of this concise and far too simplistic answer. In actuality it took approximately six years of fighting my stubborn mind before I saw the truth in these simple words. Looking back, I guess this was an encouraging way of describing the meaning of life. I mean, he could have stated that I would find the meaning of life after more years of beating myself up within vicious cycles, and in six years I would grasp a freedom from this abuse and experience true happiness through the powerful conception of self-love!

**When the heart opens,
the mind quiets and the spirit soars.**

People ask me if Ondre is my guru. He is a dear friend, and I am blessed to have him for a teacher, but I do not consider Ondre a guru because I feel it would dilute the very essence of his teachings. Ondre provides stepping-stones. He believed in me even when I had no belief in myself. Within the classes of Psychosymmetrolysis and through many daily life experiences, Ondre has passed on many tools for transformation.

We usually have a toolbox within reach, but for whatever reasons, often due to our beliefs and perspectives about certain situations, we stop ourselves from trying a new tool. The world is neither benevolent nor hostile; it really doesn't care one way or another about us. Just as one might prepare for a wilderness journey, it is up to you to take care of yourself, plan carefully, equip yourself properly, keep physically fit, use the tools in front of you and accept the consequences of your actions. PSY essentially represents a means of restoring balance, and harmony this directly leads to taking responsibility for your own life.

Do you avoid choices? Do you care one way or the other, get mind-bogged headaches or let others make choices for you? If you answer yes to any of the above, look at what you are really trying to avoid: making mistakes.

Today we are faced with more choices than ever before. The grocery store is a perfect example. There is not only standard wheat or white bread, but also bread with added soy, low carbohydrate, wheat-free, added protein, and gluten-free breads. There is whole cow milk, 2%, 1%, fat-free, chocolate, vanilla, strawberry milk, soy, rice, or goat milk. As for toilet paper, we do not have to suffer with the thin, scratchy, one-ply store brand as we once did many years earlier; we may now choose from many quality brands of plump, super-soft wiping tissue for our bums.

I had lunch at a local pizza restaurant with an elder

friend of mine. She ordered a half-cheese, half-veggie pizza and thought she had completed her order until, in a repetitively monotone manner, the cashier robotically asked, "Did you want thick, thin, skinny, herbed, or low-carbohydrate crust?" After five minutes spent on various crust explanations, and five more minutes to complete our choices, we finally sat down to wait for our exquisite skinny-crust cheese and veggie pizza.

When our pizza arrived the man dropped it heavily on the table, then smiled half-heartedly and lazily asked, "Would you like any peppers or cheese for your pizza?" My friend, with one thin eyebrow quizzically raised, stared at the man, then stared at the pizza and back again at the man, who waited patiently although a bit wearily for a reply. Shaking her head in confusion, my friend stated firmly, "There is already cheese on the pizza and many peppers too." After I explained the offering was for additional Parmesan cheese and red peppers, we had a good laugh and a good lunch.

Making choices can be fun, exciting, and an adventure for some; while for others it is difficult, vexing, annoying, and scary. Why is it scary? Because if you make a choice, it may not go the way you planned, and that makes you the person responsible for the outcome.

Making your own choices can be extremely empowering. Take a look at Helen Keller. What if she never tried walking because of the fear that she might fall? No one would know of her today. She is an incredible woman who proved that her disabilities, although challenging, would not stop her from living her life to the fullest.

> **Those most likely to overcome dangers to life and limb are people with a strong sense of personal responsibility.**

Character cannot be developed in ease and quiet. Only through experience of trial and suffering can the soul be strengthened, ambition inspired and success achieved.
—Helen Keller

Sometimes it is when we trip and fall flat on our faces, suck in a mouthful of dirt, and face challenges, that lessons learned are the most valuable. On the flip side, if you spend your time hitting yourself over the head and beating yourself up over a mistake, rather than learning from it and letting it go, most likely you are destined to revisit this situation again and again.

> **All acts will resurface and repeat until the lesson is learned and the mistake is no longer looked upon as an ugly demon, but as a helpful lesson.**

I whole-heartedly tried every avenue of perfecting perfection, assuring those around me and myself that perfection is genuinely possible; but through great disasters and humiliation, I learned that perfection is only a self-created truth that stems from the mind's imagination. And imagination, although helpful along creative paths, is only a fantasy, where we create what we want to see, rather than what is.

You could spend your days feeling sorry for yourself and envying those around you who look so fortunate with their flashing smiles, slim bodies, hefty wallets, happy family, and non-shedding dog. The truth is--there is no perfect person out there, no perfect family, no perfect partner, child, and not even a perfect dog. Although I know some will argue with me, especially regarding their dog.

We all have our idiosyncrasies, annoying habits, and mistakes. Sometimes the harder you look for perfection – in a partner or in yourself — the further away it slips. Your goal becomes impossible to accomplish because, no matter how hard you search, you will not find something that does not exist.

Melanie was only twelve when I first met her and she was already hot to be married. She talked about boys and dating when I was still more interested in playing Monopoly and reading Nancy Drew mystery books. In her late teenage years, Melanie wrote out a long, detailed list entitled "My Dream Man" in red, lusciously bold letters, which she carefully outlined in pink with an occasional flirty purple heart that saturated the limited space remaining on the parchment. As soon as a hand-some male prospect strutted her way, she whipped out the handy list and began checking off aspects that matched her dream man. Unfortunately, she was continually disappointed because no one could match her level or intensity of expectation.

Twenty years passed, along with numerous one-night stands, nine brief boyfriends, and one ex-husband. She will still say she is looking for her dream man and now admits feeling lonely. Carrying expectations to such a level that they are placed on any one person is unrealistic and can be devastating for any relationship. Worst of all, it shows the unhappiness lurking inside Melanie as she so desperately seeks to fulfill her longing for perfection from others. This is surely not a judgment about my friend or all those who suffer from this romantic delusion. I, too, once longed for this unreachable perfection.

Perfection Can Delay Action

Perfectionists, if balanced, can create magical results with what they set their mind to, but run into trouble when the perfection takes control. If this happens you will surely know, because you will find it hard to complete anything. For example, if you are writing a book, you may have the most creative story, or at least the first three chapters of it, but it will never be quite good enough for you, so you'll ask yourself, "Why bother finishing it?" Or perhaps, you always wanted to run a marathon, but first you feel that you must be in better shape, even though you already run fifteen miles every day. Or maybe you are a motivated person with a hefty list of abilities and passions, but something is stopping you from accomplishing any of them. Maybe opportunity is right in front of you, but making a decision on where to begin becomes impossible because of your desire for perfection, which can stop you dead in your tracks, or inspire you and help you move forward.

So, what is it that you always wanted to do? Maybe it's skydiving, art, woodworking, acting, or a new profession. Whatever it is for you, whether it seems big or small, stop waiting for the perfect moment to do it because, as many perfectionists are discovering, it will not come—you must go after it.

There is never a shortage of excuses such as, "I'm too tired," "I'm stressed out today," "I have PMS," "I just worked all day," or "The planets are not aligned correctly." So maybe tomorrow I will start my diet, maybe tomorrow I will start exercising, maybe tomorrow I will start to feel better. But the fact is—the time is now.

Leave nothing for tomorrow [that] which can be done today.
—Abraham Lincoln

The Burning Bush Syndrome: An Unreachable Fantasy Can Blur Opportunity

The "burning bush" syndrome is a commonly searched for and unreachable fantasy, where there may be an opening for change and growth, but the opportunity is not going to flicker flames of yellow and red until you take notice. As you drive, there won't be flashing neon signs advertising, "Stop here for unlimited spiritual opportunity." Usually, change presents itself much differently from how we expect it or want it, so it is overlooked—and when it is overlooked, the opening soon closes.

Opportunity is missed by most people
because it is dressed in overalls and looks like work.
—Thomas Edison

Stop searching for the "burning bush." The perfect opportunity is probably right in front of you! It's time to take action. You have to create the moment and go for it. Let us not only exist. It's time to begin living life—now.
Some important reminders:

- Embrace obstacles in life as lessons rather than mistakes or hardships.
- Stop dwelling in your emotions, complaining about daily tasks, and lingering in past grief or anguish. Live life, now!
- Ask yourself how any of these things can serve you.

- Take responsibility, take your life in your hands and take appropriate action to break whatever cycles continue to prevent you from truly becoming you.
- Be patient. Don't give up.
- Put a stop to the selfish "It's All About Me" mind-frame
- Stop. Look. Listen. Allow.
- Practice compassion with yourself and others, have belief in a higher being and in your own essence.

The Incredible Influence of Intent

Positive and negative thoughts are powerful and, if backed by intent, they become intensely potent. Intent can be a positive tool if you want to accomplish something or project yourself in a certain way. Setting intent means putting your mind, heart, and surrounding energy together to create a focus that can drive one to either succeed or destroy. Someone with an addiction cannot just say, "I want to stop smoking." That person has to truly want to stop, set their intent to succeed, and be ready to use the tools, work hard and achieve that goal. Someone who wants to be financially stable cannot wish it and then expect money to float from the sky. That person has to be ready to take the necessary steps and accept responsibility to make that wish a reality. Money doesn't grow on the autumn maples, and addictions do not go away overnight.

> **Achieving your intent may take some time to come to fruition. Don't give up.**

Imagination is sometimes confused with intent because, often, self-help techniques are taught to incorporate some form of visualization. If absent from intent visualization becomes your imagination creating something that is not real, and the imagination alone can become a blockage (except in the forms of art and writing.) Many visualization techniques are useful tools, but when too much imagination is combined with fear, awareness is dampened with the rising threat of a paranoid mind. In this case, awareness cannot be used properly. Instead of relying heavily on imagination, combine your visualization with intention. Do not only see the image; become it.

The way we carry and project ourselves is strengthened dramatically by our intent. Intent can be used in self-defense strikes and kicks to ensure focus and increase power upon contact. It can also be used to set personal boundaries with energy that communicates loud and clear that you are not a victim. The power of setting intent is often underestimated, but the intense results speak for themselves.

Our bodies have many pressure points, and there are two modalities we can use with them, depending on our intent. For example, acupressure helps relieve pain, balance the body, and maintain good health by gradual and steady pressure on key points on the surface of the skin. A practitioner of acupressure assists in stimulating the body's natural life force energy with the intent to heal the patient. Now let's take those same pressure points, but set our intent to restrain, harm, or disable an opponent. In the martial arts, applying pressure to these points can have a dramatic effect, causing pain and forms of manipulations. How can the same pressure points have two vividly contrasting outcomes? With acupressure the pad of the finger is used and with martial arts the tip of the finger is used, but the golden key is in the application of intent. If there is an area of your life that you would like to change and improve, each morning take a few minutes to express your intention; then follow up by taking the necessary steps to create the happiness that you deserve.

**Intentions can be used to hurt or heal.
What is your intent?**

Chapter Thirteen

The Key to Awareness:
Balancing Intuition and Logic

Awareness is simplicity itself.
—Ondre

Energetic Warning Flags

On a sweltering, muggy July morning as I walked down a quiet street in Nevada City, California, I unexpectedly felt a painful tightening in my chest, and my stomach churned in queasy knots. I quickly looked behind and around me, expecting to see something out of the ordinary, but everything seemed peacefully normal. However, I could not shake the uneasiness that was slowly consuming my body as I started to regurgitate that morning's breakfast. A miniature red flag popped up, like the ejecting jack-in-the-box clown that either scares the daylights out of you or makes you laugh at its uncontrolled wobbling. This warning flag planted deep within my solar plexus would not retire. Its persistence was not to be ignored, however irreverent it seemed to my logical mind.

Walking up Broad Street, I entered the crosswalk near the Nevada Theatre when I heard an aggressive revving of a car engine and a shrill scream of tires screeching across the pavement. An awful surge of pins and needles crossed my back. Before I registered what was happening, a cherry red car sped toward me. The driver made a left turn into the crosswalk, toward where I stood temporarily paralyzed. At tremendous speed he came at me with police cars chasing close behind. I had nowhere to run. I was trapped. *I'm going to die*, was the thought that consumed my mind. *Why now?*

Time seemed to stand still. There was a glare of sunlight on the windshield and, although the car was only a couple feet from me, there was no way to see the facial characteristics of the manic driver. Yet, even through the blinding glare, I somehow saw straight through the windshield, as if it was non-existent, to the young man who sat stiffly behind the steering wheel.

He had stringy brown hair and appeared to be about twenty. His stoned, brown eyes stared back at me, dazed and confused. We made eye contact for what seemed five minutes, but it must have been less than a single second. As we locked eyes, a peculiar feeling shot out from the top of my forehead and blasted through the windshield toward this young man. I felt sad at how lost this drug-crazed individual was and I hoped he could get help. Rather than being frightened for my soon-to-be-ending life, I felt as calm and relaxed as if I lay in a warm bubble bath with the flickering light of candles surrounding me. All this happened while the car headed full-throttle toward me, but I experienced it in slow motion.

Suddenly the man's head jerked slightly. His eyes blinked and, without explanation, his vehicle came to an abrupt halt. I jumped out of the way as it screeched through the crosswalk and squealed into the closest parking spot. Why he turned and parked, got out of the car and looked at me in complete confusion while police surrounded him, I do not know. Was it some crisis of consciousness, a soul-searching moment for him, as it was for me? Or perhaps he was merely in the devilish, soul-sucking control of the drug. The police officers pulled out their guns and yelled for me to run around the corner out of harm's way. But just as suddenly as the red car stopped, the driver suddenly appeared to realize the position he was in, and he jumped back in his car, slammed it in reverse, smacking into a police car and knocking a police officer off his feet. Down the road the car sped.

It was not until the squealing of tires and wailing of sirens were a faint whisper to my ears, that I noticed my heart beating ten times its normal rate and beads of sweat poured down my body. In the next day's paper I read that the man drove uncontrollably into a ditch after a ferocious chase. He was wanted for producing and selling the illegal drug, methamphetamine. From that day on I whole-heartedly believed in God, for there is no other explanation for how I could have survived such a close and potentially deadly disaster.

We all have warning flags. They come in all sizes, shapes, and colors. It may be a certain knowing, notion, or feeling that something seems odd, out of place. This is our awareness kicking in to remind us to take the time to stop, look around, and listen to our senses.

The warning flag is a great defense—against crime, bad relationships, or in making everyday decisions. It seems simple, yet so many people are not aware.

"Every time we face a challenge in our lives, the message is one of two things: either change and go in a new direction, or wake up. Often when people get sick, have heart trouble, problems with their bowels, or even a severe headache—it's life, their body, and the universe broadcasting: you are either in the wrong profession or the wrong place, and you need to make a change. The only problem is that we seldom listen to what we are being told.

—Ondre

A warning flag is often overlooked because, first, it is not always recognized, and, second, even if recognized, many do not pay attention to it. Why? Because often the message may be something you don't want to hear, or you think it makes more sense to trust your logical mind. We often second-guess natural, intuitive notions. When you think about it, before the information age, before the Internet, before the wide spread media, people used intuition to guide and help them make good choices. Over generations, we have exchanged something instinctively natural for a more limited, socially accepted approach to analyzing situations.

It can be difficult to listen to or even notice intuitive thoughts or "gut feelings" when your mind is consumed by the loud rumble of overloaded thoughts. Remaining calm, quiet, and clear is essential to the expansion of awareness.

A warning flag is your intuition sending you a message. It is your choice whether or not you listen to it.

The more you listen to this inner voice, the better you can hear it. The hard part is to trust an "out of the blue" thought, and act on it. If a situation does not feel right, take time to step away and look at it from a different perspective, or talk with others about it.

If you are walking down the street and a strange feeling ripples through you, whether it lasts a second or minutes, take the time to look around and take note of your surroundings. Don't be surprised if you do not notice anything out of the ordinary; you might have picked up on someone else's thoughts. Have you ever been in a public place and felt as though your personal space was invaded—like the creepy-crawlies that shiver up your spine, or the hairs that suddenly stand up on the back of your neck—but no one was close by? Perhaps someone had a happy or provocative thought about you and you picked up this thought. The good news is that you are sensitive, and this sensitivity can be used in many valuable ways to help protect you from harm. But also be aware that to be overly sensitive can shut down awareness and possibly turn into a case of paranoia.

> *Intuition is based on interpretation and, once it is opened,*
> *can easily fall prey to imagination and fear.*
> —Ondre

This is one women's story of survival through an assault, which she openly admits could have been prevented if she had only listened to her flashing intuition that encouraged her not to re-enter her van.

Trisha, 42: Nine Hours of Terror

It was still light outside at 7 p.m. on a Tuesday when I pulled into the parking lot of the bank to use the after-hours ATM. A Volkswagen "bug" was parked in front of the ATM entrance, so I waited for the driver to finish before parking my car. I left my keys in my minivan and, leaving the car running, I hopped out to make a quick bank transaction.

My back was to my car when I thought I heard something that resembled the sound of a car door closing. But after looking around, I figured it must have been something else. Returning to my car I noticed a Coke bottle on the ground outside my car's sliding door. I felt something was not right. I looked through the smoked glass windows, but saw nothing.

These inklings had entered my head and vanished in a split second, and I said to myself, "No, nothing is wrong."

I entered the car and was suddenly struck by a blow to the forehead. I was still conscious, but everything went black. I could not see or hear anything, but I felt hands grabbing at my throat. I was being choked. I tried to pull at the fingers, but I was pinned tightly against the seat. My eyesight returned and I saw cars across the street, but I could not call out. I had to keep breathing. I thought over and over: I need to breathe.

I thought that if I stopped struggling, the choking would stop, and it did. I sat limply and I heard a man's voice. "Be quiet, I'm going to pull you into the back seat, be quiet." I looked over my left shoulder and for the first time saw the man I was about to spend the next nine hours with. He duct taped my legs together and taped my arms and wrists tightly behind my back. "I am not going to hurt you; be quiet," he said. I lay on the floor below the back seats, and the man climbed into the driver's seat and began to drive fast.

My mouth remained uncovered because the duct tape did not stick on my lips and cheeks; so I spoke.

"What do you want?" I asked him. "What is your name?"

He told me he wanted the car and, after telling me his name, he asked me mine.

"Please don't hurt me; I have children," I pleaded and continued to talk with him. I could do nothing with my body, but I was calm enough to feel that I had the mental capacity to help me survive. I remember talking to Spirit and saying, "I want to live." I wondered if Spirit was going to give me an opportunity to get away from this young person who was obviously on drugs.

I felt the car go uphill and off the road. The man

tried to cross a river in my minivan but the car stopped and remained stuck in the water. I could hear what sounded like a family splashing and playing in the water. The man told me to stay low. I heard him get out of the car, and then some people tried unsuccessfully to help him push it to the other side. They finally managed to pull us back up the bank on the same side. I tried to reach a door to open it, hoping to fall out into the river and be found. I tried to climb into the back to escape. It was no use. All my attempts were unsuccessful. I would not be heard over the roar of the river anyway, except maybe by him. My cell phone sat two feet away in the front seat inside my purse, and the voices of my possible helpers slowly faded. I saw their car drive away. I was alone. My heart sank as hope of returning home slipped away.

The man came back to the car and, seeing me, he was horrified. Blood covered my face from the blow of the rock. He kept apologizing as he tried to clean me up. I said he could stop this now and not continue. I had the feeling he was cleaning me to ease his guilty conscious. When he said, "You must hate me," in a heavily nervous and agitated voice, I now felt that his intention was to do further harm to me. He asked if I did drugs. I told him I did not do drugs, but that I meditated. He questioned me about meditation and I actually led him through a meditation. Afterwards he said, "I don't know what to do. You have seen me; I have hurt you. I don't know what to do." He started touching my breasts and, after three advances, I told him I could not continue with this without being untied. I asked him if he had a condom. He pulled out a condom and untied me, while speaking to me like we were friends and again apologizing for his behavior.

"You have to take me back," I said, fearing that things were escalating, "I won't tell anybody." He told me to get in the back of the van. He forced sex on me while saying we could probably be friends.

I still did not know where we were, and it was now dark. I kept looking for any chance to escape. He cleaned the car to get rid of any evidence of blood and semen. He then sat in the front to drive, but the car did not start. He said we would spend the night here, but I reminded him that he would not want to be seen with me in the morning. He grabbed blankets out of the car and we walked for hours. Every time a car or motorcycle passed, he pushed me into the trees and bushes. I was exhausted, hurt, and had to escape.

When we stopped under a tree, I finally recognized where I was and noticed a light on in a house not far from the road. All of a sudden I was pinned against a tree, with my back facing him. I felt my pants being yanked down. He had sex with me again. At one point he turned his back to me and I took that opportunity to run. I headed for the house where I desperately hoped someone was awake. I knew that as soon as I ran from him I had lost any rapport we had, so I knew I had to be successful in getting away.

It was 4:30 a.m. when I pounded on the door and received help. I was hoping he was so paranoid about being found out that he would run the other way, and he did. I spent the next day in the ER, and the man was caught within twenty-four hours.

Although I was freed from the capture and assault, I felt vulnerable, had little energy and could not sleep for months. At first I felt like I was putting everyone around me in danger. I didn't want to be around my children because I feared I was a moving target. I was convinced at one point that the neighbors were friends with the man who hurt me. When I saw anyone with a haircut like his, I felt uneasy and unsafe. I became hyper-sensitive and a bit paranoid. Though I was labeled a victim, I was determined not remain one forever. I have all of my life to define who I am. I was not going to let nine hours define me.

After Trisha shared her story, I had the opportunity to ask her questions.

Q: What do you feel had the biggest influence in your escape?

I really had to pull together and use all my tools. The philosophy of remaining balanced and trusting in a Source higher than me—a way I attempt to live daily and teach through my yoga practice—suddenly came to the fore. My tools carried me. Staying calm, staying aware and present, even with the pain and suffering of a head injury. By staying calm, I could remember everything that took place. That helped the police pinpoint all the evidence.

Q: In what ways did you find practicing self-defense to be effective in your healing process?

At the time of the assault, I did not feel confident enough to use my body to kick or throw a punch. In the self-defense classes I took after the assault, I really enjoyed kicking, and thrusting my arms. My body was moving in a strong way even though I am a peaceful person and perhaps passive in some ways. The self-defense, along with running and racquetball, was a vehicle to help me feel my strength and power. It made me more aware, especially of the space surrounding my back. Sometimes I still feel uncomfortable in certain situations, and I ask myself, "Am I afraid that I am not safe, or am I really not safe?" I have to look with an expanded awareness.

One factor that impressed me most about Trisha was her unwavering intent to remain positive despite her shattering experience, her ability to use both intuition and logic to survive the ordeal itself, and her outlook on restorative justice. She mentioned that not only was she the victim, the offender was a victim, too.

"Everyone wants to feel powerful, loved, and connected. If they have to force someone to engage in that power, that's what they will do," she stated. This man, this attacker, offender, or whatever we choose to label him, was twenty-five years old, and had just been diagnosed with a condition that was blinding him. He had no job and had lost his driver's license; his wife was nine months pregnant, and he was told by the doctor and his family to stay on certain drugs that were making him feel high and out of control. He was sent to prison for twenty-four years essentially due to neglecting his responsibility, not questioning authority regarding the drugs he took, and for making poor decisions.

We have to look at a person's humanity. Although there is absolutely no reason to excuse his behavior, we can choose to learn from it. Restorative justice is about looking at each person involved as a human being rather than as a demon or an innocent victim. It is about having a sense of compassion and open-mindedness toward the victim and the offender.

Acquiring self-protection provides a foundation from which you act with awareness and look "outside the box." Even if threatened, self-awareness presents the mind, body, and spirit with a perspective that is flowing, nourished, and balanced.

I found myself using intuition and logic as a team during a peculiar occurrence on my way home from work one afternoon. I saw an older man in a long black cloak standing on the corner. He stood with hunched shoulders as he glanced up and down the street as though awaiting a ride. I would not have noticed him so much, but he was standing partially in the road as cars whizzed by as though he were not there. I had a strong urge to see if he needed assistance or was lost. I pulled into the bank parking lot and walked up the sidewalk as cars continued to speed by this man.

I approached him cautiously, not knowing for sure if I had made a smart move. He was definitely odd, but nevertheless, my intuition insisted it was okay. (I prayed that my intuition was accurate.) From some distance I spoke loudly, "Do you need some help, sir?" He turned to face me and when he did, I was shocked by his appearance. Although he had gray hair, wrinkled skin, and bent forward as though he were old and tired, his smile flashed a set of bright white teeth, and his eyes were a crystal blue that sparkled with youth. Met by this smile, my insides warmed, and I felt a compassion that has stayed with me to this day.

He spoke in a deep voice. "I have been waiting for you." I didn't say a word, because I saw him reach into his cloak pocket. I briefly envisioned him pulling out a gun and shooting me on the spot. My mind raced as I took note of my surroundings, the numerous ways I could disable this man, and the best way to escape--if he were to try to harm me. I was ready to spring into action when he spoke with a kind and genuine tone. "This is for you," he said. He handed me a Bible. I still felt on guard, but I took the Bible and thanked him. Before leaving, I asked one last time if he needed any assistance. The odd man did not speak to me again, but he nodded his thanks with a sagacious smile. As I walked back to my car, I turned to look once more at this curious man. Although I was only ten feet from where we conversed, when I turned around he was nowhere in sight.

Trusting intuition is important, but often the interpretation of an intuitive feeling is based on what we think it should be, not what is; for example, when the man pulled out the Bible instead of a .45 automatic. This is where silence of the mind plays an important role. The quiet mind allows true intuition to surface. The busy mind sorts through intuition with its chattering filter and dilutes or mixes the signals, which often stem from fear. If we rely only on intuition and disregard knowledge or logic, we also put ourselves in harm's way because we can miss important pieces to the puzzle.

> *"Sometimes we turn left, sometimes we turn right; our decisions direct our lives, down one path as opposed to another. Often what drives these decisions is a gut feeling or an instinct. But these things in themselves are more often than not the result of our awareness taking in and weighing up the infinite stream of information provided by our environment. The better we are at noticing, the better our instincts become. The better our instincts become, the more able we become to make good decisions."*
> —Excerpt from Rogue Warrior by John Will

Conscious self-protection and spiritual survival is an ongoing process, which transforms through truth and belief and advances through action. As this appreciation of self grows, it ripples and spreads an almighty eminence of rooted self-belief. A presence is then carried within, which clearly projects mental, physical, and spiritual flow and harmony. This activates a vital energy defense system that can deal with any situation as it arises by using both intuition and logic. This combination promotes the balance of a quiet mind and the strength of a warrior spirit, which, in turn, creates the essence—the truth, the core—of self-defense: *whole body/mind consciousness.*

We all have the potential for being a murderer. What stops some and encourages others? The difference lies in the degree and choices of our actions. A murderer or crime assailant uses anger against another person by inflicting pain and hurt through demoralizing, raping, or killing. Others use anger to hurt themselves through food, drugs, alcohol, etc. As individuals, we have the ability to deprive ourselves of success, self-belief, and happiness.

The process of Psychosymmetrolysis stimulates the range of awareness potential that you and others possess—both negative and positive. It provides the ability to see situations for both the good and the bad, and with the knowledge and faith that all things happen for a reason. Where there is good, there is evil; where there is love, there is hate; where there is light, there is dark. The contradictory nature of our world, and way we live, intertwines within the universe and its cycles. There is truly a flip side to everything. Our bodies can be strong, healthy, and vibrant, while at the same time vulnerable and weak. The body, mind, and spirit have the potential to defend or attack.

The only battles are the ones being fought within. Take it out of you and challenge the world. Help make it a better place-no kind act is too small. This is natural healing.
—Ondre

It is not how awful the situation we are in that determines the outlook on the rest of our life. It is our *perspective* and *interpretation* of a situation that can either lead to danger or promote growth and healing. The choice is always ours.

REFERENCES

BOOKS, MAGAZINES, STUDIES

ABC World News, Serial Killer Profiles Often Inaccurate, February 2005.

Cook, Philip and N. Cohen, *Abused Men: The Hidden Side of Violence.* Greenwood Publishing Group, Westport, CT, 1997.

Hatsumi, Masaaki, *The Way of the Ninja.* Kodansha International, LTD, Tokyo, Japan, 2004.

Hoban, Jack, *Living and Thinking as a Warrior.* Chicago, IL, 1988.

Kellerman, Arthur, "Men, Women and Murder," *The Journal Trauma*, July 17, 1992.

Mayor, Jerry & John P. Holms, *Bite Size Einstein*, St. Martins Press, New York, NY, 1996.

Merriam-Webster Dictionary, Springfield, MA, 2004.

Richelson, Jeffery, *The U.S. Intelligence Community*, Westview Press, Boulder, CO, 1999.

Kurr, Stephan, *How to Bodyguard Yourself,* Opsec Intelligence, Las Vegas, NE, 2002.

Tjaden, Patricia & Nancy Thoennes, Findings from the National Violence Against Women Survey, November 1998.

Vorpagel, Russell & Joseph Harrington, *Profiles in Murder: An FBI Legend Dissects Killers and Their Crimes*, Perseus Books, Cambridge, MA, 1998.

INTERNET RESOURCES

http://www.ojp.usdoj.gov/bjs/cvict.htm
Bureau of Justice Statistics Crime and Victims 12/10/07

www.feminist.org/other/dv/dvfact.html 4/19/07

http://apps.nccd.cdc.gov/PASurveillance/DemoComparev.asp
CDC Division of Nutrition, Physical Activity and Obesity U.S. Physical Activity Statistics 1/23/08

www.fastdefense.com
excerpt from Rogue Warrior by John Will 12/19/07

www.endabuse.org 5/05/07

http://www.cdc.gov/mmwr/preview/mmwrhtm/mm5526a1.htm
2/03/08

www.add-adhd-help-center.com/depression/statistics.htm
10/1/07

www.teenadvice.about.com—emergency.com/roofies.htm
8/16/07

Resources: Pass it on

*Internet sources are subject to change

PYCHOSYMMETROLYSIS/HEALING

Ondre Raymond/Natural Healer
Devoted entirely to spiritual growth and empowerment.
www.ondre.com

Advanced Botanical Research
Founded on the belief that in nature there are the tools that can help heal; first they must be found and then applied.
www.advancedbotanicalresearch.com

INTERNET RADIO

Open Mind Entertainment Network (OMEN)
A community-based world broadcast dedicated to creating a global network of inspiration, hope, and healing.
www.openmindradio.com

SELF-DEFENSE INSTRUCTION

Safety Awareness Training
A multiple level approach to personal safety
www.lilareyna.com

NATIONAL HELP HOTLINES

National Domestic Violence Hotline
1.800.799. SAFE 1.800.799.7233

Help is available 24 hours a day, 365 days a year. Assistance is available in English and Spanish with 140 languages through interpreter services. Hotline advocates are available for victims and anyone calling on their behalf to provide crisis intervention, safety planning, information, and referrals nationally.

National Teen Dating Abuse Hotline (NTDAH)
www.loveisrespect.org

A 24-hour national web-based and telephone helpline created to help teenagers 13-18 experiencing dating abuse.

The Rape, Abuse, Incest National Network (RAINN)
1.800.656. HOPE

Helpful advocates transfer callers anywhere in the nation to their nearest rape crisis center. It can be used as a last resort for people who cannot find a domestic violence shelter in their area.

Connecticut Sexual Assault Crisis Center (CONNSACS)
1-888-999-5545

A national clearinghouse for information and resources for victims of sexual assault.

Child Help USA National Child Abuse Hotline
1.800.4. A.CHILD

Multilingual crisis intervention, providing referrals to local service groups, and offering professional counseling on child abuse.

Day Care Complaint Hotline
1.800.732.5207

National Child Abuse Hotline
1.800.25.ABUSE

Boys Town Suicide and Crisis Line
1.800.448.3000
Counseling for parent-child conflicts, marital and family issues, suicide, pregnancy, runaway youth, physical and sexual abuse, and other issues.

National Association of Anorexia Nervosa & Associated Disorders (ANAD)
847.831.3438

National Mental Health Association
1.800.969.6642

Cancer Information Service
1.800.422.6237

Elder Abuse Hotline
1.800.252.8966

National AIDS Hotline
1.800.342.2437
Information and referrals to local hotlines, testing centers, and counseling.

Nationally Sexually Transmitted Disease Hotline
1.800.227.8922

Poison Control
1.800.362.9922

Missing and Exploited Children
1.800.843.5678

National Cocaine Hotline
1.800.262.2463
Information, support, treatment options, and referrals to local rehab centers for all types of chemical dependency

Alcohol Hotline Support and Information
1.800.331.2900

National Adolescent Suicide Hotline
1.800.621.4000

Covenant House Hotline
1.800.999.9999
Crisis line for youth, teens, and families.

BOOKS

Martial arts
Be Like Water: Practical Wisdom from the Martial Arts by Joseph Cardillo, Warner Brothers Inc., 2003.

Martial Arts Mind and Body by Claudio Iedwab & Roxanne Standefer, Human Kinetics 2000.

The Spiritual Practices of the Ninja by Ross Heaven, Destiny Books, 2006.

Domestic Violence
Ending Intimate Abuse: Practical Guidance and Survival Strategies by Albert R. Roberts & Beverly Schenkman Roberts, Oxford University Press, 2005.

Abused Men: The Hidden Side of Domestic Violence by Philip Cook, Praeger Publishers, 1997.

The Verbally Abusive Relationship: How to Recognize it and How to Respond by Patricia Evans, Adams Media Corporation, 1992.

Sexual Assault
The Rape Recovery Handbook: Step by Step Help for Survivors of Sexual Assault by Aphrodite Matsakis, Raincoast Books, 2003.

139 Ways College Women Can Prevent Sexual Assault by Richard Hart, Verum Publishing, 2006.

Depression
Feeling Good Handbook by Dr. David Burns, Penguin Group, 1999.

The Beast: A Journey Through Depression by Tracy Thompson, Penguin Group, 1996.

The Mindful Way Through Depression: Freeing Yourself From Chronic Unhappiness by J. Mark G. Williams, John Teasdale, Zindel Segal & Jon Kabat-Zinn, Guilford Press, 2007.

Eating Disorders
French Toast for Breakfast: Declaring Peace with Emotional Eating by Mary Anne Cohen, Gurze Books, 1995.

Overcoming Bulimia Workbook by Randi E. Ph.D. McCabe, Traci L. Ph.D. McFarlane, & Marion P. Ph.D. Olmstead, Raincoast Books, 2003.

Anorexia Nervosa: A Guide to Recovery by Lindsey Hall & Monika Ostroff, Gufze Books, 1999.

Mental Illness

Creating Mental Illness by Allan V. Horwitz, The University of Chicago Press, 2002.

50 Signs of Mental Illness: A Guide to Understanding Mental Health by James Whitney Hicks, Vail-Ballow Press, 2005.

Nutrition and Mental Illness: An Orthomolecular Approach to Balancing Body Chemistry by Dr. Carl C. Pfeiffer, Healing Arts Press, 1987.

For Parents of Children/Teenagers

How to Really Love Your Teenager by Ross Campbell M.D., Chariot Victor Publishing, 2003.

Talking to Tweens: Getting it Right Before it Gets Rocky with your 8-12 year old by Elizabeth Hartley-Brewer, Da Capo Press, 2004.

Addictions

Addiction: Why Can't They Just Stop? by Susan Cheever, John Hoffman, Susan Froemke, & Sheila Nevins, Rodale Press, 2007.

Addiction: A Personal Story by Lacy D. Enderson, Bennett Deane Publishing, 2006.

Personal Growth/Inspiration

A Course in Courage: Disarming the Darkness with Strength of Heart by Gates McKibbin, Ph.D., Field Flowers Inc, 1998.

Laughing Buddha, Crouching Uncle: Zen and the Art of Comedy Improv by Robert Smith, Live Long Laugh Loud Publications, 2008.

Spirit Animals by Victoria Covell, Dawn Publications, 2000.

Are You Really Too Sensitive?: How to Develop and Understand Your Sensitivity as the Strength It Is by Marcy Calhoun, 1987.

Leading Like Madiba by Martin Kalungu-Banda, Double Storey Books, 2006.

Messages From Above by E. Nonymous, Intuitive Development Publishing, 2004.

Health and Wellness
Acu-yoga by Michael Reed Gach & Carolyn Marco Matzkin, Japan Publications, 1981.

Why Zebras Don't Get Ulcers-An Updated Guide to Stress Related Disease and Coping by Robert M. Sapolsky, Henry Holt and Company, 1994.

Loving What Is by Byron Katie & Stephan Mitchell, Three Rivers Press, 2002.

Internet Safety
Safety Monitor: How to Protect Your Kids Online by Mike Sullivan, Bonus Books, 2002.

Look Both Ways: Help Protect Your Family on the Internet by Linda Criddle, Microsoft Press, 2006.

Personal Safety
Travel Can Be Murder: The Business Traveler's Guide to Personal Safety by Terry Riley, Applied Psychology Press, 1994.

How to Bodyguard Yourself by Stephan Kurr, OpSec Intelligence, 2002.

The Complete Guide to Personal Safety and Home Safety: What You Need to Know by Robert L. Snow, Da Capo Press, 1995.

- Personal Notes -

About the Author

Lila Reyna founded Safety Awareness Training in 2001, a life-changing self-defense program for adults, teens and children. Trainings and events involve themes and content similar to those included in the book. Lila is a speaker, radio show host, and martial arts instructor. She strives to pass on her passion to create and live a life of balance, motivation, and heightened awareness.

Lila resides in Northern California with her husband and children.

You can join Lila weekly on the
Open Mind Entertainment Network
www.openmindradio.com

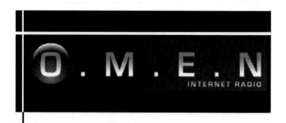

O.M.E.N is an internet broadcast company dedicated to bringing entertainment and information to a world audience. Offering diverse shows not normally aired on mainstream radio, O.M.E.N. is celebrated for its support of independent musicians and broadcasters.

O.M.E.N., the world's resource for fresh and innovative programming, giving voice to new thought and perspectives.

Open Mind Entertainment Network
www.openmindradio.com
Changing the world
one computer at a time.

**If you enjoyed the book, check out the
FREE Self-Defense for the Mind, Body, and Spirit
NEWSLETTER
Sign up today at www.lilareyna.com**

WHAT OTHERS ARE SAYING

"Lila's instruction is an amazing mind-opening, confidence building, practical experience in the art of personal safety. The techniques I learned were simple and effective, and the group exercises helped me move from a mindset of victim to a woman of empowerment."

—*Mary Larson, California*

"I thought self-defense was all about kicks and punches. While fending off an attacker is an important skill, learning how to prevent a potentially dangerous situation is an even greater tool. It was exhilarating to see the changes in myself and classmates' demeanors as seeds of self-belief and awareness were firmly planted and ready to grow."

—*Carol Moore, Hawaii*

"Safety Awareness Training not only stimulates your awareness, it creates a bridge to the physical, mental, and emotional bodies. This class allows people to take charge of their lives, to become empowered, physically become stronger, mentally be more alert to their surroundings, and finally, to reconnect emotionally. For me, it has helped define better who I am; allowing me to believe in myself again."

—*Carolyn Story, Arizona*

"The workshops are fun, informative, and an inspiration to people of all ages. Awareness is the foundation of self-defense and Lila empowers individuals to find a sense of themselves."

—*Angie Trathen, California*

To send correspondence to the author of this book, or for more information about Safety Awareness Training seminars and speaking engagements in your area visit www.lilareyna.com.